FEELING BETTER

FEELING BETTER

THE
6-WEEK
MIND-BODY PROGRAM
TO EASE YOUR
CHRONIC SYMPTOMS

(Previously published as *Stop Being Your Symptoms
and Start Being Yourself*)

ARTHUR J. BARSKY, M.D., AND
EMILY C. DEANS, M.D.

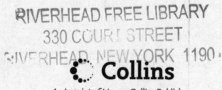

Collins
An Imprint of HarperCollinsPublishers

Originally published in hardcover by Collins, an imprint of HarperCollins Publishers, in 2006 under the title *Stop Being Your Symptoms and Start Being Yourself*

First Collins paperback edition published 2007

Designed by Jeanette Jacobs

Library of Congress Cataloging-in-Publication Data is available upon request.

ISBN 978-0-06-076614-6 (pbk.)

06 07 08 09 10 11 ID/RRD 10 9 8 7 6 5 4 3 2 1

To our patients

Contents

Acknowledgments————

We would like to thank a number of individuals who have provided invaluable help in bringing this book to completion. Dr. Linda Schmidt was instrumental in conceiving the project in the first place. William Phillips lent us his clear vision and trenchant suggestions. Our editor, Gail Winston, provided a steady hand and experienced guidance throughout the process. Brettne Bloom, our agent, gave us unerring advice and counsel from beginning to end. We'd also like to thank our families for their assistance and support throughout the long and sometimes (for them) tedious process. Finally, of course, we are indebted to our patients, who have taught us much of what we learned and tried to present here. We thank you all.

Foreword

Do you suffer from ongoing pain or other chronic medical symptoms, including fatigue, acid indigestion, eczema, and migraines? Do they interfere with your family life, your daily routine, or your work to the point where you are looking for answers and help? Have you been forced to give up activities in your life, or find that the symptoms get worse under stress? Do you worry about your symptoms more than you'd like to?

In this book, you will learn how to control your symptoms instead of letting your symptoms control you. The book is divided into three parts. Part 1 is an introduction and is intended to help you know a little about us, the authors. After all, wouldn't you be reluctant to listen to a doctor's advice if you didn't know the doctor? Part 1 also helps set the stage for the six-week program to learn new ways to think about and react to your symptoms. In Part 2, we present the six sessions that make up the program of "Stop Being Your Symptoms and Start Being Yourself". Part 3 teaches you several general principles for coping with chronic symptoms and illness, and gives broad guidelines for living well.

We suggest that you first scan the book through from cover to cover, without paying too much attention to the details, just to get an overview of our program. Then go back and read Part 1 before you begin the six-week program in Part 2. You should read each of the six chapters in Part 2 one week at a time. During the weeks between chapters, do the homework and the exercises you just read about, in order to put the material into practice and prepare you for the next chapter. Continued practice and further understanding of the principles given in this book will help you live well despite your symptoms. In Part 3, we give you some guidance about maintaining a healthy lifestyle and conclude with some final thoughts about the lessons learned from people who cope successfully with illness.

FEELING BETTER

PART ONE

*A New Way to Think
About Symptoms*

CHAPTER ONE

Introductions

Emily C. Deans, M.D.

My mother has allergies. She wakes up in the morning with puffy eyes and headaches. Sometimes she has to sit in a dark room with a cold towel on her forehead. She coughs, sneezes, and speaks with a hoarse voice. Occasionally her allergies cause nausea. She bends over a humidifier; she uses nose sprays and antihistamines. In the past, some of the sprays made her nose bleed. Another medication made her blood pressure shoot through the roof. Another one gave her hives, and she had to send me to the store for some emergency Benadryl. She has had the air ducts of the house cleaned, and her pillowcases are mite-proof. She avoids the outdoors. Her carpets are shampooed religiously. She tests her sinuses in the morning by pressing on them before putting on her makeup—she can determine the amount of discomfort she will feel the rest of the day by how much this hurts. Her allergies have everything to do with her quality of life, and dozens of doctors and medications over the years have done very little to help.

My mother's allergies are a big part of why I became a doctor. I had, of course, an interest in science and a desire to help out, but at the heart of my motivation was finding something to help my mother. This book is for her.

This book is also for Jack Heresford. He was a veteran in his mid-thirties, married with a baby girl, whom I met as a medical student in a neurology clinic. He had terrible headaches that started in the back of his neck and crawled up the muscles into his scalp. He couldn't stand bright lights or reading. Sometimes he couldn't even drive. He tried migraine medicines and mild pain medications and was starting on the heavy-duty ones like Percocet and fentanyl, but nothing helped. My professor at the time, an attending neurologist, said there wasn't much we could do for him.

"They're tension headaches, Emily."

"But they're ruining his life."

"They're classic tension headaches." The neurologist shrugged, content with his diagnosis. In truth, Mr. Heresford had undergone a number of tests to prove he wasn't that sick. We knew he didn't have a brain tumor or high blood pressure or an aneurysm. From the neurologist's point of view, Mr. Heresford should have been happy that the headaches were not a sign of any "serious" disease— they were serious enough to disrupt his entire life, but not serious enough to kill him. I've thought about Mr. Heresford many times in the years since, wondering if he still goes back to the neurology clinic, collecting his pain medication prescriptions, and what his life is like now.

I don't remember every patient I've met. Fairly early on, though, maybe during the first hundred, I discovered that a large percentage of people who come to the doctor don't have serious, life-threatening medical illness. They have osteoarthritis, back pain, migraines, muscle aches, allergies, fatigue, insomnia, chronic sore throats, chest discomfort, heartburn, trick knees, abdominal pain, and intermittent constipation or diarrhea. Since you are reading this book, I'm willing to bet you've suffered some or most of these ailments in your lifetime, some intermittently, some ongoing. You may have missed work, school, exercise, or social activities because of these symptoms. Like my mother, you may have spent thousands of dollars on medical care and alternative therapies to help. This book is for you.

For much of my medical training, I learned how to differentiate between the serious and the not-serious. I learned that what was important was not to miss the things that might kill a person. Treatment plans involved ruling out heart disease, cancer, or infection. Once we doctors can rule these illnesses out, we are happy.

Our patients, however, are not. They may be relieved, understandably so. But they are still left with the discomforts and pains. Sometimes their lives are ruled by these "mild" illnesses, like my mother's, and they come back to the doctor seeking help. And what I learned in medical school was that there wasn't all that much doctors could do for these chronic symptoms. I didn't learn much of anything that could help my mother or Mr. Heresford.

I decided to do further training in psychiatry after medical school. I figured if I couldn't help my mother's sinuses from overproducing, at least I could learn how to help her deal with the stress her condition caused. But psychiatry training, I soon found, followed the same basic tenet as the rest of medicine: Rule out or treat the serious diseases—schizophrenia, bipolar disorder, major depressive disorder, and other conditions that lead to disability or death. There may be more emphasis in psychiatry on quality of life and the patient's experience than in other medical fields, but even so the main goal is still to diagnose and treat "serious" disease. Obviously, there are very good reasons for this focus. However, I still didn't find much I could do to help my mother.

Two and a half years into psychiatry training, I had a few more tools to help my mother with her stress, but I still couldn't address the heart of her problems. To be honest, I had given up looking. In the long journey through medical school and residency training, I lost sight of my original goal.

Then I attended a lecture given by Dr. Arthur Barsky, one of my supervisors at the Harvard Longwood Psychiatry Residency Training Program, and a world expert on how medical symptoms are related to the mind. During this lecture he presented the results of a landmark, five-year study he had done under the auspices of the National Institutes of Health and Harvard Medical School. He presented the data, methods, and results of his study, and by the end of the lecture I was so delighted I could barely sit still. Finally! I had learned something that could help my mother, Mr. Heresford, and everyone else with ongoing "benign" medical symptoms.

For decades, Dr. Barsky had been searching for the same answers I had been looking for. He had developed a six-week behavioral program that used mind-body techniques to address just such symptoms as backache, insomnia, fatigue, allergies, and ongoing noncardiac chest discomfort. He created a treatment plan to help cope with and diminish all those benign, chronic symptoms for which there was not much doctors could do. Then he spent five years proving that it worked.

To find patients to help him demonstrate that his new methods were effective, he sent out more than 6,000 questionnaires to patients in primary care clinics at Massachusetts General Hospital and Brigham and Women's Hospital, both in Boston. Not surprisingly, he got a lot of phone calls from patients and doctors who were frustrated with what traditional medicine offered them. He also put advertisements in the subways and buses in Boston recruiting into the study anyone who was having trouble coping with symptoms that medical treatment had failed to alleviate. He received hundreds of phone calls.

He studied a group of 187 of these respondents. Approximately half the patients underwent his treatment in six individual therapy sessions along with their usual medical care. The other half continued with their regular medical care but did not undergo any therapy. All the patients completed a research interview when they entered the study, and underwent the same interview six and then twelve months later.

The treatment was found to be beneficial: when compared to the outpatients who did not receive the treatment, those who did had fewer and less intense bodily symptoms, spent less time thinking about their health, were less concerned about their illness, had a better health-related quality of life, and had less disability and impairment in their daily activities. These benefits were significant, and continued six months and then a year after treatment had ended.[1]

During the lecture I attended, Dr. Barsky reviewed the basic components of each of the six behavior modification sessions used in his study. He used cognitive behavioral techniques—known to most people as "mind-body" medicine—and focused on medical symptoms. As he described each component of the treatment, I became more and more convinced that his work needed to be shared with people other than the doctors in training, social workers, and faculty that made up the audience of his lecture. It needed to be presented in a form that anyone could pick up and learn. It needed to be presented in a book!

I thought of Mr. Heresford and my mother and the hundreds of people riding the subway, too frustrated or frightened about their symptoms to seek help. How much suffering could be relieved if people just had access to the proven system Dr. Barsky developed? What if primary care physicians finally had a resource they could give their patients who suffered from benign but chronic and bothersome medical symptoms? These thoughts emboldened me to approach Dr. Barsky during a supervision session. After hearing my ideas, he agreed to write this book with me. Thus with great pride and pleasure, we present the simple six-week treatment to you. It is a treatment without medications that can be learned in less than two months, has no side effects, and costs nothing outside the purchase price of this book, some writing paper, and a pen.

Arthur J. Barsky, M.D.

When we first met for supervision, Emily asked me how I had become interested in the relationship between medical symptoms and the mind, since it is not an area that has received much scientific study. Psychiatrists have mostly focused on disorders such as depression and schizophrenia that are obviously psychiatric in nature. Internal medicine physicians, for their part, are trained to detect and treat anatomical or physiological abnormalities that cause recognized diseases. Their *initial* focus is generally not on their patients' discomfort, disability, or difficulties in coping with their disease, but rather on the disease process itself.

Yet what surprised and interested me most in medical school was the obvious gap or disconnect between the two. The physical disease process that concerns the doctor and the patient's personal experience of feeling sick are often very different. Simply treating the disease all too often does not cure the discomfort and distress. While some patients with very serious medical conditions manage to cope remarkably well and find that their symptoms are tolerable, others with the very same disease feel much sicker and have a much harder time of it. Their symptoms are worse, they are more disabled by their condition, and it seems to take over their lives. The patients with good coping skills, in contrast, maintain a positive outlook, are able to minimize their symptoms, and manage not to let their symptoms rob their lives of meaning and pleasure.

Some patients have no serious medical disease that we can detect with a test or an examination, but suffer with symptoms that make them virtual invalids. Early in my professional career, I met Peggy Hampton. She was a gifted graphic artist, a terrific tennis player, and she had a keen sense of humor. Toward the end of her (very successful) college years, she developed a bad case of bronchitis. Although it cleared up promptly with antibiotics, she was left feeling weak and worn out. Everything she did, from buying a birthday present for a friend to preparing a meal, seemed to require a superhuman effort and left her exhausted afterward. Yet a series of competent specialists could find "nothing wrong"—no evidence of lingering infection, no problems with her hormones or metabolism. In the doctors' terms, Peggy was a normal, healthy specimen. But fatigue was ruining just about every aspect of Peggy's life. She turned down a promising promotion at work because she feared she wouldn't feel well enough to undertake the travel it would entail; she was afraid to meet men and go on dates because she knew she would eventually have to disclose her illness and was sure they would then lose interest in a long-term relationship with her. Her illness had become the most important part of her existence, a defining personal characteristic. She no longer just *had* her symptoms—she *was* her symptoms. And her illness became a way to explain to herself why her career was going nowhere, why she was lonely. She was an invalid—yet from her doctors' viewpoint, "nothing at all was wrong."

In contrast, there are other people who are able to cope with horrific diseases, and manage to live full and satisfying lives despite them. When their doctors look at their X-rays and blood test results, they consider them to be very sick, victims of progressive or chronic diseases. Yet from the patient's perspective, their sickness is only a small part of who they are, of how they feel about themselves and the lives they lead.

I also had the good fortune of meeting Alison Moore. She had developed rheumatoid arthritis as a youngster, and by the time she was in her late thirties, she had become physically disabled. She had to stop working as an accountant, and found that simple daily chores like opening jars and buttoning her blouse were difficult without assistance. Yet Alison did not let these realities erode her sense of herself as a competent, effective, useful, and helpful person. As she was forced to give up tasks that required physical dexterity, she found other things to do that allowed her to express what she most valued about herself, which was her ability to be helpful to others. Though she had to stop working full time, she was able to spend more time in volunteer and community activities such as raising money for the public library and organizing a neighborhood watch association. Since she remained cheerful and continued to see herself as competent and helpful to others, she was an attractive person to be around; she found many who admired and liked her and were happy to help her out when she needed it. In contrast to Peggy, Alison was considered very sick by her doctors, but managed to preserve a meaningful, rewarding, and pleasing life.

I couldn't help but wonder about the differences

between Peggy and Alison. What was it about them that made them respond to illness so differently? What were Alison's secrets? How was she able to deal so well with illness? She and others like her obviously had a great deal to teach us.

These questions seemed so important that I decided to focus my professional career on them. I chose to specialize in psychiatry because I thought that the answers must lie in the psychosocial realms of personality, attitudes, behavior, and personal relationships. Psychiatry seemed to offer the best vantage point from which to understand these areas. The psychiatrist is privileged to come to know people in a deeply personal way, to ask about their fears and wishes and commitments and regrets. He or she is able to hear what people think and feel when they are ill, how they persevere and struggle with their illness, what frightens and depresses them, and what they try to do about it. It must be in this personal realm, I thought, that the answers to successful coping are to be found.

After finishing my psychiatric training, I specialized in consultation psychiatry, which is the subspecialty area of psychiatry that deals with the overlap of medical and psychiatric disorders and treats patients who have psychological difficulties as a result of their medical illnesses. Over the more than twenty-five years since, I've worked with many medically ill patients who are suffering psychologically as well as physically, investigated the relationships between psychological forces and bodily symptoms, and taught medical and psychiatric trainees like Emily. I've discovered how much you can learn from your patients if you ask them what works and what doesn't work, help them to cope with pain and disability, encourage them to unburden themselves, and listen to what they have to say. Some of them express their reflections in such simple and wise phrases that you never forget them.

A number of years ago I treated a young woman afflicted with cystic fibrosis. She lived her entire life in the shadow of that disease; she knew that even with the best of medical care, her life would be shortened. Yet she somehow came to terms with this situation, was not angry at her unjust fate, and continued to care about and for those around her. When I told her what a wonderful job I thought she was doing in such difficult circumstances, she responded that she had learned to accept her situation. She said that for her it all came down to truly *accepting* the existence of her illness and the limitations it imposed, to being able to say to herself, "I want it but I know it's not for me." That insight, so simply and beautifully stated, is full of wisdom.

So the credit for much of this book goes to patients like these, who can teach the rest of us how to accept our situations and overcome chronic symptoms, compensate for them, minimize them, and keep them in perspective. As Oscar Hammerstein wrote, "When you become a teacher, by your pupils you'll be taught." Over the years of working with ill patients and studying the process of adapting to illness, a number of principles, observations, and insights emerged. I used these observations in my clinical work and in my teaching and then gathered them together into a formal treatment program. Along with my colleagues at Harvard Medical School and the Brigham and Women's Hospital in Boston, I tested this treatment program in a careful, large-scale, research study. The results confirmed my clinical impression that patients did indeed find the program helpful. Having completed this study, I felt more confident about suggesting our ideas and guidance to a wider audience.

But I never thought about how this program could be made accessible directly to the public until Emily suggested in that supervisory session that we put the material into a book for a general audience. As we talked the idea over, it made more and more sense to me: the treatment manual we used in our research could indeed be presented in a book that could reach many more people than we could hope to reach in clinical practice.

About This Program

All the people in the research study for this program received complete medical evaluations for their symptoms. It is crucial to remember that, throughout this book, we are only talking about symptoms for which you've already sought medical attention, and for which either your doctor could not find a serious medical cause or has treated them but the symptoms persisted nonetheless. Our program is not a *substitute* for a thorough medical evaluation and appropriate medical treatment, but rather is an *adjunct* to them.

Millions of people—fully one-third of the people who visit the doctor every year—have legitimate aches, pains, and troubles that do not fit under the current medical definition of "serious" or life-threatening illness. These are people who suffer but have not been treated satisfactorily by modern medicine. No one alive goes without medical symptoms altogether, but with this program, you can change how you react to symptoms, feel about them, and think about them. In so doing, you will learn how to control your symptoms rather than letting your symptoms control you.

CHAPTER TWO

Your Health Belongs to You

Before we outline the six-week program to stop being your symptoms and start being yourself, it is important for you to see the bigger picture—that you are not alone in living with symptoms that resist medical treatment, continue to distress you, and erode the quality of your life. Many Americans face the very same problem, and the suffering these symptoms cause seems to have been worsening over the last few decades. In this chapter we will examine how social, historical, and psychological forces can make your bodily symptoms more troublesome. Armed with this knowledge, you will then be in the best position to take advantage of the six-week program that follows. You can take control of your health, rather than being a prisoner of symptoms.

Doing Better and Feeling Worse[1]

DOING BETTER

Modern medicine has astounding powers to detect and cure disease, powers hardly imaginable just a few years ago. We have techniques to open clogged arteries and reverse heart attacks. We can reattach severed limbs and surgically correct fetal heart malformations while the fetus is still in the womb. We have created artificial skin and hearts, kidneys and cartilage. Tiny cameras can be swallowed to photograph the inside of the stomach and intestines. Special viruses have been modified so that they can insert new DNA to replace the faulty genes that are responsible for some inherited diseases.

As a result of all this progress over the last fifty years, the death rates from most major killers, including heart disease, stroke, and several forms of cancer, have declined dramatically. Deaths from heart disease have fallen by 40 percent since 1970. Breast cancer mortality is 20 percent lower than it was in 1990. AIDS is no longer the imminent death sentence that it once was, and patients routinely live comfortably for more than a decade following the diagnosis. According to all the major indices of collective health, we are indeed an extraordinarily healthy society. Life expectancy is at an all-time high, and the gaps between men and women and between whites and blacks are narrowing. The average American lived 47.3 years in 1900, 68.2 years in 1950, and an astonishing 76.9 years in 2000.

These exciting triumphs over lethal diseases, however, have had a perverse effect: they make our everyday ailments seem worse.[2] Medicine's new therapeutic powers have actually made it harder to live with the less severe, chronic illnesses that continue to defy medical science. We can save premature babies who are born no bigger than the size of your hand, but we still can't prevent children from getting recurrent ear infections. We can characterize the microscopic, cellular changes that come with aging, but we can't prevent the dry skin and the insomnia that accompany it.

Our astonishing medical advances serve to underscore our more limited progress against chronic illnesses, degenerative disease, aging, and the wear and tear of daily life. Do you suffer from migraines? Lower back pain? Ever miss a day of work due to premenstrual pain or allergies or heartburn? Despite medicine's conquest of many diseases, you know from personal experience that plenty of illnesses remain to afflict us. We need only think of ourselves or our families, our neighbors or our coworkers, to realize how prevalent are fatigue, asthma, osteoarthritis, constipation, memory problems, and the like. These are all conditions that are indisputably real, but can prove very resistant to medical treatment.

Despite the best medical care, these symptoms continue or recur, and can come to play too prominent a role in our lives. They're uncomfortable, distressing, perhaps embarrassing; they impair our leisure activities, sex lives, social plans, or productivity at work. In one typical survey, 86 percent of the respondents reported having at least one bothersome symptom.[3] Fatigue, for example, is among the most common and troubling of symptoms. In survey after survey, between 17 and 19 percent of adults report being bothered by "prolonged," "substantial," or "chronic" fatigue.[4] Lower back pain is another ailment so common among us as to be almost universal. A full 80 percent of us have been troubled by back pain over the course of our lifetimes, and 25 percent of us have experienced it in the recent past.[5] In fact, one of the most difficult parts about studying treatments for back pain is finding experimental control subjects who have never had back pain! You are certainly not alone in struggling with chronic symptoms that modern medicine can't cure outright.

These symptoms are serious enough to prompt medical attention. In 1998 there were 61.3 million doctor visits for colds and sore throats alone, and only 61 million visits for high blood pressure, diabetes, and coronary heart disease combined.[6] All of this doctoring occurs despite the common knowledge that a cold will get better in a week if you go to the doctor—and will last seven days if you don't.

How can we be doing better and feeling worse? This paradox is partly the result of medical progress itself. Many of the diseases that used to cause sudden or untimely death—such as pneumonia, tuberculosis, and childhood infections—can now be prevented or cured. But our medical progress has been more limited when it comes to chronic diseases and the frailties that come with a longer life. Thus the people saved from premature, early death due to infections, strokes, and heart attacks now live long enough to develop Alzheimer's disease, arthritis, and cancer. While the odds of surviving a heart attack have vastly improved, the survivors are often left to struggle with angina or congestive heart failure, conditions that produce chronic symptoms and disability that can't be cured outright or treated away.

So the result of these medical advances is that while they enable us to live longer, the *proportion* of life spent in ill health has actually *increased*. Our dramatic gains in lifesaving treatments have *increased* the proportion of people living with chronic ailments. Dementia is a vivid and omnipresent example. The incidence of dementia is rising because we can now treat the pneumonia, kidney failure, and heart attacks that used to end people's lives before they grew old enough to become demented.

The term "failures of success"[7] describes this phenomenon, in which some diseases actually occur *more* often in the population, rather than *less* often, as a result of medical advances. The failure of success simply reflects the laws of statistics. Put bluntly, if you avoid dying from a heart attack, your chances of getting cancer are going to increase.[8] It is like Russian roulette: reducing the chances of one cause of death obviously and inevitably increases our chances of succumbing to another. And if the ultimate cause of death is a more chronic and more symptomatic condition, then the prevalence of symptoms has actually gone up. And, all this time, little has been done to help our long-lived population cope with these ongoing illnesses.

FEELING WORSE

Depressing evidence from a number of sources suggests that Americans are increasingly bothered by their symptoms and chronic ailments, more disappointed with their medical care, and more dissatisfied with the state of their health.[9] This is evident in polls and surveys, in the skyrocketing rates of disability, and in the massive flight to alternative and complementary medicine.

Large nationwide surveys reveal that the proportion of us who believes we are in poor or only fair health has risen steadily, from 13.4 percent in 1993 to 15.5 percent in 2001.[10] Likewise, the number of days per month that we report feeling physically unhealthy—days in which our "physical health [was] not good"—has risen from 3 days a month in 1993 to 3.5 days a month in 2001.[11] Thus, we seem to be more troubled by our symptoms and more distressed by nagging ailments than were previous generations.[12]

We are also increasingly disabled by our symptoms, as evidenced by workers' compensation claims over the past thirty years. Musculoskeletal pain is now the single most frequent reason for long-term sickness compensation and permanent worker disability.[13] While there was no increase in the incidence of verifiable injuries and demonstrable back disease (such as herniated discs or bone spurs) between 1964 and 1994, the number of disability claims for lower back pain increased by fourteen times the growth of the population during that same period.[14] Currently, of all the workdays lost to sickness, more than half are due to symptoms without physical evidence of major illness or injury.[15] Also, the average number of days off from work per episode has increased,[16] indicating that we are more disabled by our symptoms than we used to be.

The growing dissatisfaction with medicine's inability to treat chronic symptoms is evidenced in the increasing use of alternative and complementary medicine. Americans visit these practitioners most often for chronic symptoms—such as headaches, digestive problems, and neck pain and stiffness—that have defied conventional medical treatment, rather than for very serious or potentially fatal conditions like cancer, diabetes, and strokes.[17] More than 42 percent of American adults used an alternative therapy in 1996. (The most common forms were relaxation therapy, massage, chiropractic, and energy healing). But only six years earlier, the comparable figure was 33.8 percent.[18] In 1997, there were more visits to complementary and alternative healers than to primary care doctors![19]

The Difference Between Symptoms and Disease

Why are we fleeing from Western medicine, with its focus on disease, to alternative forms of treatment that have a more holistic emphasis? Perhaps it is because Western medicine has a fundamental flaw when it comes to the cause-and-effect relationship between disease and symptoms. Symptoms can be produced by more things than physical disease; they can be produced by our life experiences, expectations, beliefs, and emotions.

The Roman philosopher Epictetus said, "Man is

disturbed not by things, but by the view he takes of them."
Your perception of an event can be just as important as,
or even more important than, the actual event itself. The
perceiver creates the world he or she perceives. Remember the last time you saw a magnificent sunset? What was
it like for you? Did you get a sense of exhilaration, beauty,
or nostalgia for past sunsets that were equally lovely? The
sensory stimuli that entered your brain—the external
sensations you perceived—were nothing more than light
waves. But your total conscious experience of beauty or
nostalgia or exhilaration was something you created in
your head. You embellished those light waves with emotions, fantasies, memories, and associations that all together created your personal experience of the event.

The same thing happens with bodily sensations.
Your experience of pain, for example, is more than a matter of damaged tissue causing pain signals to travel to the
brain. The total conscious experience of pain depends
on what the painful sensation means to you and the circumstances you are in at the time. Your beliefs, hopes,
knowledge, and worries about the painful sensation all
shape how the pain feels. At times these even make it possible to experience the sensation of pain without much of
the suffering and anguish that would normally accompany it. Good examples of this are the pain that comes
with extreme athletic exertion (such as successfully com-
pleting your first marathon), or the pain of childbirth.
Pain can occur without as much suffering or agony when
the painful experience brings people closer to a long-
cherished goal.

Your conscious experience of pain is composed of
two separate and distinct elements. There is the painful
sensation itself, with its characteristics like location, intensity, and duration; and there is the unpleasantness or suffering dimension—the thoughts it triggers, the memories

it evokes, the threats it signifies, the anxiety it arouses. Some patients receiving narcotics for severe pain become aware of this distinction when they notice that while the drug has alleviated their discomfort, the painful sensation remains. These patients often say, "I can still feel the pain, but it doesn't bother me now."

There are two distinct neural pathways underlying these two dimensions of pain.[20] One pathway leads up the spinal cord to a pain center in the brain (called the somatosensory cortex) that enables us to identify and locate the pain. But the pain signals are also relayed to another center, the anterior cingulate cortex, in a different part of the brain. Here they are integrated with input from other brain areas where emotions, memories, and associations reside to produce the quality of discomfort and unpleasantness that accompanies the pain. A recent experiment was able to distinguish these two dimensions. Subjects were given a hypnotic suggestion to decrease the unpleasantness of an experimentally induced pain while they underwent a brain scan.[21] The hypnotic suggestion decreased the *unpleasantness* of their pain but did not alter their ratings of the *intensity* of the pain. The brain scans done at the same time showed that the hypnosis lessened the neural activity in the cingulate (the part of the brain that integrates the sensation with thoughts and emotions), but did not lessen the brain activity in the somatosensory cortex (the part of the brain responsible for perception of the stimulus).[22]

This distinction between the sensory dimension of a symptom and its unpleasantness means that symptoms and disease don't have a fixed, one-to-one relationship to each other. Disease is an abnormality in the structure or functioning of the body; symptoms are the personal, psychological experience of disease. Disease and symptoms are not the same thing, and modern medicine is designed to treat disease, not symptoms. It is possible to have troublesome symptoms without a serious medical cause, and it is possible to successfully treat a serious disease without curing the patient's symptoms. Fortunately, it is also possible to improve many symptoms without curing the underlying disease that causes them.

Lower back pain, the second most common reason for visiting the doctor, illustrates this distinction perfectly.[23] As many as 90 percent of patients with severe lower back pain have perfectly normal spine X-rays. On the other hand, one-third of healthy people *without any complaints of back pain* actually have bulging or ruptured spinal disks when x-rayed with CAT or MRI scans.[24] Heart palpitations illustrate the same point: most people bothered by palpitations do not have any serious heart rhythm irregularities, and most people with serious heart arrhythmias do not complain of palpitations.[25]

Many severe and even disabling symptoms are not accompanied by any serious pathological process that can be identified with Western medicine's current diagnostic tools. Physical exams, blood tests, and even advanced body scans can't pick up the cause of innumerable symptoms. Among all the patients going to doctors because of a bothersome symptom, no serious medical explanation can be found in *one-third* of the cases![26] When patients waiting in their doctors' waiting rooms are specifically asked if they've been bothered by any of a long list of symptoms, 75 percent or more of all the symptoms that they complain of are never found to have a serious medical basis.[27] Yet these medically unexplained symptoms can be just as distressing and disabling as the symptoms resulting from a demonstrable medical disease. Worse, many of these unexplained symptoms continue for long periods of time. And with no "disease," there is no "cure."

Many people with severe, recurrent chest pain have normal cardiac tests—that is, exercise stress tests and X-ray examinations of their coronary arteries fail to detect anything wrong. But the absence of serious heart disease does not mean that these patients' chest pain is either trivial or short term. Although their rates of heart attack and cardiac death remain low, they have persistently high levels of pain at work, in social situations, and in their daily activities, and they make many visits to the doctor. Indeed, the amount of disability they experience is comparable to that of patients who have heart attacks and diagnosable heart disease.[28]

Even when doctors do find a disease present, the symptoms accompanying that disease are unpredictable and variable: two persons with the identical disease can have two very different sets of symptoms and two very different personal experiences of that same disease. Arthritis patients have been widely studied in this respect, and a number of studies show that their pain is not closely linked with the extent of the damage in their joints as measured with X-rays.[29] One patient, Freda Wilkes, continues to golf in spite of two hip-replacement surgeries. Her husband, David, who needed only one hip replacement, is so impaired that he needs Freda's help in order to bathe and get dressed.

Among patients with asthma, laboratory tests of lung function are poor predictors of how much breathlessness they report.[30] Similarly, in men with benign enlargement of their prostate gland, urinary symptoms are not closely related to laboratory measurements of urinary obstruction.[31] When patients complaining of insomnia spend the night in a diagnostic sleep laboratory, little relationship is found between their complaints of not being able to sleep and the actual recordings of their brain's electrical activity during the night.

With these facts in mind, it may not be surprising to learn that successful medical treatment of a disease does not guarantee symptom relief. For example, a new therapy for rheumatoid arthritis was found to be very effective in reducing inflammation as measured with blood tests, but it failed to relieve the patients' pain and stiffness.[32] In a study comparing antacids with an inactive pill for the treatment of ulcers, the active medication produced greater ulcer healing than the placebo pill but was no better in relieving their symptoms.[33] Similar findings have been seen in treating anemia: significant improvements in the patients' blood counts were not accompanied by reductions in symptoms such as headache, dizziness, and fatigue.[34]

We've just seen that it is possible to treat a disease successfully without the symptoms going away. But even more important for our purposes is the fact that *it is possible to relieve symptoms without curing the underlying disease.* The powerful placebo effect is a striking illustration of this. Placebo pills—pills that the pill-taker believes are an active medication but that are in fact composed entirely of an inactive substance—have been shown again and again to relieve the symptoms of a wide variety of diseases, such as asthma, depression, high blood pressure, and ulcers. Overall, roughly one-third of patients experience significant symptom relief from taking a placebo pill, even though the placebo itself is not reversing the disease process.

Doctors, Patients, and Medical Care

Modern medicine assumes that diagnosing and then treating disease will cure symptoms. Doctors are taught in medical school that tissue destruction or damage leads directly and inescapably to a characteristic set of symptoms. But as we have just seen, symptoms are not all that closely linked to those disturbances of tissue structure and function that we call disease. Your experience of symptoms, even very bothersome, persistent, and disabling symptoms, doesn't map neatly onto your physician's ability to diagnose and treat disease. And this gap between medicine's concept of disease and the patient's experience of symptoms must be bridged when a doctor can't find a disease to treat, or if the symptoms persist despite treatment. The symptoms, not just the disease, must be addressed.

Medical education emphasizes physical sciences like biochemistry, anatomy, and physiology, and doctors are not as well trained to deal with the personal experience and the psychological aspects of illness. So they are often poorly equipped to alleviate their patients' symptoms by helping them deal with their fears, beliefs, expectations, and feelings. (It brings to mind the old adage about education that "It takes many years of training to learn to ignore the obvious.") Though physicians want to be helpful, they often find that they don't know how to be. They grow disillusioned and frustrated with this part of their job, so they try to minimize it or ignore it. Patients can sense their doctor's growing frustration, which compounds their distress and only makes the situation worse.

A vicious circle has thus been created, in which the physician's frustration causes patients to feel more hopeless, which only discourages the physician further, and the cycle repeats itself. Some doctors will place the blame squarely on their patients and label them as "crocks," "turkeys," or hypochondriacs, hinting—or in some cases actually suggesting—that it is "all in their heads." The patients, of course, end up feeling much worse.

This failing of medical care is often compounded by

the mistaken assumptions many patients harbor. We tend to assume that medicine, with all its scientific advances, is capable of diagnosing and treating all of our ailments. If doctors can transplant a human heart and program a robot to do brain surgery, surely they can cure simple headaches or that unpleasant ringing in your ears. And if we believe that medicine should be able to cure everything, then patients whose symptoms are not cured conclude that their doctors must not be taking them seriously enough or simply don't care enough about their case to get to the bottom of their problem. Worse, perhaps the doctor is ignoring the symptom because he or she believes it is "imaginary" or "all mental."

The only solution is to help patients and doctors alike to understand the processes that go into perceiving and experiencing symptoms. This book breaks down and examines these processes, then describes how to use symptom perception to begin to feel better instead of worse.

Why We Differ from Each Other

We have seen that two people with the same ulcer or the same inflamed knee can have very different levels of discomfort and suffering. Why?

First of all, the sensory nervous system varies from person to person. Just as some people have sharper vision or better hearing than others, some people are more sensitive to what is going on inside their bodies.[35] These people, called by the medical profession "symptom amplifiers," are more aware of their hearts beating, their pulse throbbing in their ears, hunger contractions in their stomachs. Their symptoms are more severe and intense than other people's. And they are often bothered by symptoms such as throat tickles or mild aches that nonamplifiers aren't even aware of at all.[36] This characteristic is quite stable over time, and seems to be hardwired into our nervous systems.

Second, some people have more intense symptoms than other people because of their upbringing. When we are young, our families teach us how much to focus on our symptoms, how much to worry about them, how much to give in to them and curtail our activities because of them. There are many everyday examples of this. If a child arrives at the breakfast table and announces that he can't go to school because he has a test that morning, his mother will still make him get on the school bus when it arrives. But if a child in another family (or that same family) announces at the breakfast table that he can't go to school because he has a stomachache, he is far more likely to be allowed to stay home. In this way we teach children how much to focus on the physical or the psychological symptoms of stress and anxiety. These two children will more than likely grow up with different levels of symptom reporting. Did your family pay a lot of attention to your symptoms when you were sick as a child? How alarmed and worried did they become? How quick were they to keep you home from school or march you off to the pediatrician? These sorts of experiences can create a general tendency to monitor one's symptoms and to experience them as more severe and more significant.

Third, our own experiences with medical illness in childhood can shape how sensitive we are to symptoms and how much they bother us. Adults who were seriously or chronically ill when growing up tend to be more aware of symptoms and more alarmed by them than those of us who never had serious health problems when we were young.

You can't change these factors. You can't change how your brain is wired, or what your childhood experiences were, or the way you were raised. But there are a number of other factors that make us more symptomatic that we *can* control and change. It is these factors that the six-week program targets. But before we actually begin the program, we need to learn something about the psychology of symptom perception and see how the contemporary American culture around us can make it more frustrating and difficult to live with chronic ailments. It is important to understand how these social and psychological forces influence you, so that you can use them to your advantage rather than allowing them to make things worse.

The Psychological and Social Forces That Make Symptoms Worse

Just how healthy or how ill we feel depends a lot on our personal psychology. How else can we explain the fact that many seriously ill people are actually relatively satisfied with their health status? Although very sick people such as quadriplegics do have lower levels of general well-being than people who are not sick, many do not suffer as much as outside observers expect them to.[37] Sixty-eight percent of people with severe, disabling disorders say they are somewhat or very satisfied with their lives. (Ninety percent of people who are not disabled respond "somewhat satisfied" or "very satisfied" to the same question.) How is it that severely ill people—for example, those with cancer—report their satisfaction with life is only somewhat worse than that of nonpatients?[38] Conversely, how can we explain that many people who are not seriously ill are plagued by disabling symptoms, are dissatisfied with their health, and experience poor health-related quality of life?

Two very important psychological factors determine how much our illnesses bother us and how satisfied we are with our state of health: our *expectations* about how healthy or ill we should be; and the health of those to whom *we compare ourselves*. In general, our satisfaction with a situation depends in large measure on what we think that state of affairs *should* be. If I expect a C on a final exam in college, I'm delighted when my actual grade is a B. On the other hand, that exact same B is met with dismay if I thought I deserved an A. This is a general principle—that our beliefs and expectations about how things should be will influence our contentment and satisfaction with how things actually *are*.

How healthy we've been led to expect we should feel influences how healthy we actually do feel. The discomfort that we mistakenly expected to be cured is more distressing than the discomfort that we always knew was unavoidable and would just have to be put up with. Suppose you need to have knee surgery for arthritis, and your surgeon has said, "You'll be good as new!" When you are left with some residual pain and stiffness, you may be disappointed, and perhaps even depressed and bitter. But if your surgeon was more cautious, telling you about the possibilities of a less than perfect outcome, the exact same result might seem satisfactory, and you probably won't be nearly as upset or angry. When we have been misled into believing that an infirmity is curable, it becomes more difficult to endure when it isn't. Disillusionment compounds the physical distress and heightens your dissatisfaction.

Satisfaction with our jobs and our financial state, and even our overall level of happiness, is shaped by our expectations. For example, how content people are with their income and their material standard of living depends in large measure on how wealthy they thought they would be at this point in their lives, and on the life-styles of those around them. How wealthy you feel depends not just on how much money you have, but on how much you expected to have and how much your friends and neighbors have. This applies to self-esteem as well: the self-esteem of students of *equal* ability differs depending upon the ability of their classmates. Students in poorer schools where many of their classmates do poorly have higher self-esteem than comparable students at higher-quality schools where their relative class standing is lower.[39]

Your distress and dissatisfaction with your health are relative and are determined by comparing yourself to some standard—that is, to some imagined ideal of how healthy you should feel. So when it comes to coping with chronic symptoms, whom you compare yourself to influences how you feel. Symptoms that are ubiquitous within a group of people are often not even recognized as symptoms. For example, in some poverty-stricken and disadvantaged groups where almost everyone has diarrhea, respondents to health surveys do not report diarrhea as a symptom; since almost everyone has it, it is not perceived as abnormal or a reason for seeking medical attention. In the same sort of way, your tolerance for that annoying, persistent cough you have right now depends on your reference point: If you compare yourself to the robust ideal of vigor and fitness portrayed in a TV commercial for a home treadmill, you feel lousy; but compared to an uncle wasting away with chronic lung disease, you feel well off. The second type of comparison is called a "downward comparison,"[40] and makes us feel better about our own health.

We view our own situation in a more favorable light when we become aware of others who are in more difficult situations and confronted with worse problems. In a psychology experiment, for example, the presence in the room of a physically handicapped person increases the subjective well-being ratings of the experimental subjects.[41] As people learn to cope with serious illness, they begin making downward comparisons—that is, they compare themselves to people who seem sicker or more disabled than they are. In so doing, they come to appreciate that things could be worse. Breast cancer patients have been found to go through this process of downward comparison as they learn to cope more successfully with their disease.[42]

In a study of patients with rheumatoid arthritis, those who made downward comparisons were judged to be coping better with their condition.[43] Each time Deborah Wilkins comes to the hospital for treatment of her advanced arthritis, she feels encouraged; she always notices "someone who is blind or in a wheelchair in the lobby or in the waiting room—someone who is a lot worse off than I am. It seems like my situation really isn't that bad."

On the other hand, when we make "upward comparisons" with people who seem *better* off, our sense of well-being declines and we become more dissatisfied with our own situation.[44] Comparing yourself to someone who appears to be healthier or more fortunate than you are highlights your own limitations. How good do you feel about your lifestyle when you watch television shows about the fancy cars, beautiful clothes, glorious vacations, and elegant houses of the rich and famous? Though you may be quite comfortable in your living situation, it is always possible to have more luxuries and creature comforts. Recognizing this can help you keep perspective and appreciate what you have. Just watching the hype on television—not only about health, but about what constitutes success and happiness—can leave you feeling sick and unsatisfied.

Social and Cultural Forces

Trends in contemporary American society aggravate our distress and make coping with symptoms more difficult.[45] They influence our personal psychology by heightening unrealistic expectations and supplying idealized images of good health, coaxing us into making upward comparisons. This in turn amplifies symptoms and makes them harder to live with. We are not a nation of self-centered, self-indulgent, complaining hypochondriacs. Rather, our rising distress over our symptoms and growing difficulty coping with them are being fueled by powerful societal and cultural forces. Understanding how these forces contribute to feelings of ill health is a vital part of learning to cope with and take more control over how you feel and help you in developing strategies to feel better. Knowledge is power—in this case, the power to recognize where and when you are being influenced in negative, unhelpful ways.

Americans today are indoctrinated through television, media, movies, and even by medical institutions, with unrealistic and idealized expectations about health and medical care. We are led to believe that good health should be a state of almost perfect physical well-being, devoid of all bodily distress, without any physical impairments or limitations. We are told that modern medical science can confer upon us a state of "wellness"—a state of robust and youthful vigor, ageless beauty, and corporeal bliss.[46] We are in effect being coerced into constantly making upward comparisons. Such idealized views of health and unrealistic expectations of medicine inevitably lead to disappointment when we contrast them with the reality of daily life, with its sometimes liberal doses of allergies, memory lapses, insomnia, and stiffness. When it turns out that many of our nagging symptoms and chronic conditions cannot simply be treated away, they become even harder to bear. Living with migraines, eczema, fatigue, allergies, and angina is difficult, but it is even more difficult when we have been told that medicine can cure it all and are led to expect a lifetime free of distress.

Our standard for judging good health has been elevated so much that we are now more bothered by symptoms and infirmities that in the past we were able to tolerate better.[47] Because we expect medicine to deliver complete well-being, we feel resentful when it turns out that all our aches and ailments can't be cured. It is as if an implicit promise has been broken, that there is something fundamentally unfair about a chronic ailment that persists despite medical attention and our having deliberately and conscientiously lived a "healthy lifestyle." We almost feel as if we've been cheated out of something we were entitled to. Surely our persistent symptoms must result from medical negligence, environmental pollution, governmental or corporate malfeasance, or personal failure.

The Profit Motive

Total health care expenditures in the United States reached $1.6 trillion in 2002, between 13 and 14 percent of the gross domestic product. The profit motive has led to the growth of a giant "medical-industrial complex"[48] that stimulates and then satisfies consumer demand for health-related products and services. From the business perspective, nagging symptoms, infirmities, and ailments represent a vast potential market. Advertisers, manufacturers, entrepreneurs, and professional groups all promote the fantasy that any symptom, any physical imperfection, any dysfunction, can be cured with the right product or service. Health is viewed as a commodity that can be purchased, medicine has become a business, and the medical care system is now an industry.[49]

Sophisticated marketing plays on the universal wish to live a symptom-free life. We are told that we don't have to put up with dry skin, baldness, or acid indigestion because a remedy is at hand. All you need to do is flip on the television at any hour to catch an infomercial peddling a product or service that may in fact have maximal fantasy fulfillment but minimal effects.

This enormous, for-profit health care industry includes propriety hospitals, investor-owned diagnostic laboratories, emergency and walk-in services, freestanding imaging facilities, dialysis units, and ambulatory surgery centers. They view themselves as businesses, competing for a share of the market with aggressive public relations and marketing campaigns. It is estimated that they garner one-quarter of the total amount of money spent on personal health care.[50] Hospitals have been among the quickest to commercialize, undertaking massive marketing and advertising campaigns.[51] They boast elective surgery at convenient hours and entice customers with gourmet food and free transportation. They have opened retail shops and catering services, and even offer frequent-user bonuses patterned after the airlines' frequent-flyer programs.[52]

But the problem is that all this marketing raises our expectations to a level that ultimately can't be met.[53] Those of us who find we are not citizens in this supposed symptom-free utopia of "wellness" are disappointed, and discover that now our symptoms seem even worse by comparison.

Medicalizing Nondisease States

Another trend that amplifies our symptoms has been termed "medicalization." This refers to a historical trend in which ailments and maladies that we previously had to accept as facts of daily life have been progressively redefined as diseases that can be treated medically.[54] Many of the conditions that are being medicalized can indeed be treated successfully, to the enormous benefit of those afflicted with them. But at the same time, medicalization also heightens our expectations to an unrealistic degree about the conditions that are not fully treatable, and this makes them less tolerable and more distressing.

We now have medical treatments for undesirable or unattractive physical characteristics that were not previously thought of as diseases, such as baldness (hair transplants), short stature (growth hormone treatments), nearsightedness (LASIK surgery), and facial wrinkles (Botox injections). Antioxidants and vitamins are prescribed to reverse the physical decline that accompanies normal aging. We consult doctors in order to improve our performance at work and in the classroom (with drugs for attention deficit disorder) and on the athletic field (with steroids and stimulants). Though we have always had "trouble sleeping," only recently have "sleep disorders" entered our lexicon; insomnia used to be a condition we simply endured, or for which we tried a favorite folk remedy or drank a highball before bedtime. Now, however, we diagnose the problem in specialized sleep disorder clinics. Something similar has happened with sexual performance: sexual dissatisfaction and not being "in the mood" have been transformed into sexual "disorders," to be cured with sex therapy and Viagra.

With cosmetic surgery, physical features that are simply unattractive or undesirable have become medically and surgically alterable, so they now seem like disfiguring deformities. Cosmetic surgery patients are not "sick"; they may have physical characteristics that are unwelcome or unattractive, but they do not have a disease. The purpose of cosmetic surgery is to make us satisfied, not well. But there is a problem: medicine can never cure physical unattractiveness—no matter how many cosmetic procedures we undergo, some of us will always be more attractive and younger-looking than others.

The history of medicalization reveals a consistent pattern. Medical interventions that were initially developed to treat clear-cut diseases were gradually applied to less and less severe variants of that disease until they came to be used on people formerly thought of as normal. The treatment of short stature illustrates this historical progression. Growth hormone therapy was initially developed to treat children with abnormally low levels of growth hormone. But over time its use was broadened to include children who do not have an endocrine disorder but are simply shorter than their peers.[55] But again there is a problem: no matter how many children we treat with growth hormone, some children will always be shorter than others.

A similar progression has occurred in sports medicine, which was originally developed to treat injuries resulting from athletic exertion, but then broadened its mission to include the enhancement of athletic performance in perfectly healthy individuals with steroids and autologous blood transfusions and stimulants. But again there is a fundamental problem: there is no replacement therapy for the lack of athletic ability. Likewise with geriatric medicine, which evolved from its initial goal of diagnosing and treating the diseases that accompany longevity into attempts to alter the normal aging process itself. But surgery can't arrest the passage of time.

Medicalization has unquestionably alleviated genuine suffering and benefited many afflicted people who could not have been helped before. Our point is *not* that we have failed to alleviate many of these newly medicalized miseries and ailments; quite to the contrary, we can now ease many forms of suffering that were formerly incurable. Rather, it is precisely because these successes are so substantial that they create the expectation that everything that ails us is potentially curable, that there are no limits to what biomedicine can achieve, that whatever troubles us about our bodies or our performance can be successfully treated away. Medicalization fosters an unattainable ideal of symptom-free lives. This fantasy in turn leaves us more dissatisfied with the remaining symptoms and dysfunctions that resist treatment. The more we equate physical health with total well-being, the more pervasive illness becomes.

The Mass Communications Media

The mass media are another societal force that amplifies chronic symptoms and heightens dissatisfaction with them. Their portrayals tend to alarm us about the significance of every twinge and ache, while at the same time they exaggerate the therapeutic power of medicine's latest advances, promising more than can realistically be delivered. The media repeatedly draw your attention to every imaginable discomfort you might have, and suggest that while it may well be serious or even deadly, it can be treated almost miraculously. And if it's already being treated, then they suggest that the treatment itself may be dangerous or potentially fatal (think of Celebrex, Viagra, or hormone-replacement therapy). The sheer volume of medical bulletins and health warnings is overwhelming, from television medical correspondents and full-length documentaries, to medical spots on the radio, to newspaper columns on health. The "Health and Medicine" sections of our bookstores swell with each passing month, and a whole new generation of magazines devoted exclusively to health now beckon from every newsstand. The nightly news is suffused with alarms, advice, and warnings, from the latest tally of West Nile virus or SARS victims to the risks of Ebola, mad cow disease, "flesh-eating" bacteria, bird flu, and Lyme disease. Should you ignore your indigestion when the last television episode of *ER* featured a character whose "heartburn" turned out to be a heart attack?

In the hunt for instantaneous, "breaking" news, the media also tend to exaggerate the potential benefits of still unproven research—resulting in so-called "medico-media hype."[56] Preliminary studies of highly experimental therapies are too often portrayed as established treatments that promise immediate relief for sufferers. These early findings may be trumpeted as definitive, providing unequivocal answers that will immediately lead to practical treatments. This morning's report about plaques found in the brains of aging laboratory mice is supposed to result in a pill to help a senile parent this afternoon. The media tend to focus on a single positive study while ignoring a sea of negative ones. For example, a 1995 study published in the *Journal of the National Cancer Institute* prompted the *New York Times* headline "New Study Links Abortions and Increase in Breast Cancer Risk," when the manuscript actually contained the caveat that *forty* previous studies found no such association.[57] The supposed link between electromagnetic fields and cancer furnishes an example of the media's treatment of medical news:[58] While a large French study found *no* such link for twenty-five of twenty-seven types of cancer (the exceptions were for two extremely rare types of leukemia, for which the associations were weak and inconsistent), the study was reported in the *Wall Street Journal* under the headline "Magnetic Fields Linked to Leukemia."

This hype unrealistically heightens our expectations and leads to confusion and disappointment when the overstatement (or misinformation) ultimately becomes evident. The net result of all this is to amplify symptoms that resist treatment and make them seem more ominous, worrisome, and distressing.

Vested Interest Groups and Disease-Specific Constituencies

A multitude of special-interest groups and disease-related constituencies have arisen over the past few decades. These include advertisers, advocacy groups, insurance companies, and even physicians and medical institutions themselves. While they can have a beneficial effect, they can also promote an unrealistic view of medicine's diagnostic and curative power and an idealized standard of good health. In furthering their mission, clamoring for public support, and lobbying for funding and governmental or legislative attention, they can heighten our expectations (and our anxiety) excessively.

These groups broadcast their message to the public at large, as is exemplified by drug company advertising and the advent of diagnostic testing on demand. In television commercials and print advertisements, pharmaceutical companies suggest that you don't need to tolerate any symptom or dysfunction, because a cure already exists for it. You need only "ask your doctor" for the miracle pill that will bring you "relief"—relief of headaches, constipation, coughs, impotence, premenstrual cramps, high cholesterol, and dozens more.

A related development has come with the rise of do-it-yourself diagnosis, that is, patient-initiated laboratory testing. Diagnostic tests that could formerly be obtained only through a physician are now available on request. Walk-in CT scanning centers, for example, provide total body scans on demand (for over $1,000), without any medical indication whatsoever. At the local drugstore you can engage in the so-called "private practice of medicine" by purchasing at-home medical testing kits for diabetes, infertility, cholesterol, HIV, hepatitis, and urinary tract infections. Rather than having to go to your doctor to decide whether particular laboratory tests are medically indicated, you can now obtain even the most sophisticated tests yourself over the Internet. (One Web site offers a choice of 5,600 such tests, for example.)

Physicians, hospitals, and researchers themselves have at times oversold the public on their powers and promised more than they can deliver. Among some medical institutions and physicians, professionalism has given way to entrepreneurialism,[59] and in advertising and self-promotion they may exaggerate the benefits of their services. Hospitals, for example, tout new specialty programs to deal with every imaginable ailment or complaint, from noninvasive brain surgery to "spine centers" to liposuction. But too often they promise more than they can reasonably deliver.

The Deteriorating Doctor-Patient Relationship

With clinical medicine's increasing subspecialization, reliance on technology, and pressure for productivity, doctors have less and less time to listen to patients, to support and comfort them. Sarah Leeson, a patient with carpal tunnel syndrome, complained that her doctor failed to consider her as a whole person. "He treats me like a hand," she remarked. A doctor's personal attention, encouragement, concern, and guidance are among the best ways to help patients cope with symptoms that can't be cured medically. But this takes time—time that many doctors no longer have.

Distrust of medical authority is growing. More people now rely on friends and relatives as their main source of health information.[60] With the rise of managed care and HMOs, many worry that doctors' financial incentives are in conflict with patients' best interests. The physician-patient relationship that was once characterized by trust and confidence is being replaced by a business relationship whose motto is, increasingly, "buyer beware."[61] In extreme instances, physicians come to be viewed as the problem rather than the solution. When doctors lack a diagnostic explanation for severe, bothersome symptoms, the physicians themselves are sometimes held responsible for the patient's continued suffering. Dr. Allan Steere, the world's foremost authority on Lyme disease, has questioned the scientific validity of the Lyme diagnosis in chronically symptomatic patients who have no laboratory evidence of harboring the Lyme bacterium. However, many of these patients, convinced that they have a chronic form of the illness, have done more than disagree with the doctor—they have vilified him. They've physically threatened and harassed him, and accused him of "destroying" them.[62]

Nowhere is the deterioration of the physician-patient relationship more evident than in the rising tide of medical malpractice suits, which have tripled in the last ten years. Malpractice insurance costs doubled in a single year (2001), and premiums for obstetricians in Miami, Florida, run as high as $200,000 per year. The soaring costs of medical malpractice have resulted in the closure of maternity wards and trauma centers and left entire communities without any practicing neurosurgeons.[63] The point here is not that physicians have suddenly become less competent than they were, but rather that our *expectations* of them and of the outcomes of medical care have changed. Behind the skyrocketing medical malpractice actions lies the fantasy that all ailments are curable, all adverse outcomes preventable. Malpractice litigation often results from the frustration of unmet expectations of medical care, the unrealistic expectation that every condition is diagnosable and treatable. If any distress or disability persists after medical treatment, someone must be at fault.

In the past, the doctor-patient relationship provided the solace, support, and comfort that are so helpful in coping with chronic ailments and refractory symptoms. But the deterioration of this relationship has eroded doctors' power to heal. This means that physicians are now less able to palliate their patients' symptoms, to reassure and comfort them about their illnesses, and we have an even harder time handling our symptoms than we once did.

Who Controls Your Health?

It is becoming more difficult to cope with the chronic ailments and symptoms that resist treatment. This is not our fault, nor is it a reflection of our own poor coping abilities, nor the result of personal weakness. Rather, it comes from historical, societal, and cultural pressures that play on our personal psychology by excessively heightening our hopes and expectations. It becomes so much harder to cope with conditions that can't be cured when we were led to expect that we wouldn't or shouldn't have to face them in the first place.

Recognizing these pressures is the first step to coping better with your symptoms. You can see through the unrealistic come-ons, the marketing and the hyperbole, to acquire a more realistic understanding of health and illness and learn how to overcome chronic and distressing symptoms. We aim to help you take back control over your thoughts and feelings about your health. Your health does not belong to society, television, special interest groups, entrepreneurs, pharmaceutical companies, the Internet, or even to your doctor. It belongs to you.

PART TWO

Feeling Better: The Six-Week Program to Stop Being Your Symptoms and Start Being Yourself

CHAPTER THREE

Week 1—Shift Focus from Your Symptoms to Yourself

The six-week program begins now. Each of the next five chapters takes the mind-body factors that shape how you experience your symptoms, explains them, and supplies you with hundreds of strategies to decrease your symptoms. The sixth and final chapter in Part 2 brings together all the concepts you will learn and guides you in making a plan to keep using your new skills. Read each chapter at the beginning of the week, then practice the exercises in each chapter for the rest of the week. Then go on to the next chapter. The time and work you will spend in the next six weeks has a specific and achievable goal—to take control away from your symptoms and give it back to you, where it belongs. Remember, this program has been scientifically tested, and it works!

Attention and Distraction

The attention you pay to a troubling symptom is one of the most important factors in how you perceive it. The more you concentrate on an unpleasant or uncomfortable sensation, the worse it becomes over time. Don't believe this is true? Concentrate for a moment on your throat. Although it wasn't bothering you before, you might now notice a tickle. You might respond by clearing your throat, but that doesn't seem to help. As you continue focusing on your throat, now it starts to feel scratchy and dry. You may even end up coughing.

Many symptoms are the same way. Have you ever observed a group of people talking and noticed that if one of them coughs or yawns or scratches himself, others in the group are soon doing the same? The initial culprit calls everyone else's attention to a trivial itch or a tickle that they did not notice before. Now, as they attend to the sensation, it becomes bothersome, and they do something to try to relieve the discomfort.

The psychologist James Pennebaker[1] studied this phenomenon. He had a group of people watch a movie and provide minute-by-minute ratings of how interesting it was. Then he played the same movie for a different audience and observed when people coughed. Sure enough, their coughing occurred during the most boring parts of the film. At those points, they were less absorbed in what was happening on the screen and most likely to notice a mild or otherwise unobtrusive bodily sensation. Another of his experiments involved two groups of joggers. One group listened to bits of distracting conversation (the sort you might hear while riding in an elevator) through a set of headphones while they jogged on the treadmill. The second group heard the sounds of their own labored breathing. Although the two groups had the same heart rates, blood pressures, and respiratory rates, the second group felt more fatigue, palpitations, and sweating.

This same phenomenon was demonstrated using dental patients who had just undergone tooth extraction.[2] Half of the patients were asked to rate their pain every twenty minutes for two hours following the surgery.

The other half were only asked for a single pain rating two hours after the surgery. The first group reported much greater pain at the two-hour point than the second group did.

These findings can be explained by the predictable cycle involved in symptom amplification. It begins with noticing a particular symptom followed by an apparent increase in intensity of the sensation. Now, because the symptom seems to be worsening, you begin to worry that it might be more serious. This alarming idea causes you to pay more attention to the symptom, to focus and concentrate on it more. But doing so only makes you note subtle changes and distinctions in the symptom that didn't seem to have been there before. The more you concentrate, the more the pain might seem to be spreading, or throbbing more, or becoming sharper. It will seem as if the problem may be growing or worsening. If you think the symptom is caused by a disease, these added sensations make you suspect that the disease is advancing or worsening or is more severe than you originally thought. Naturally, your anxiety gets worse, and more and more attention is devoted to the symptom. The cycle goes round and round, with you caught up in a vortex of anxiety and symptom amplification.

Consider the case of Jim Reyering:

Jim's father died of a heart attack early in the summer. About a month later Jim was helping his brother move a heavy bureau when he developed a tightness across his chest. He felt nervous and wondered if he might be having a heart attack, so he started to really concentrate on everything going on in his chest. The more attention he paid to the tightness, the worse it became. Then it felt as if his heart seemed to be speeding up and pounding harder, and it seemed to be getting more difficult to catch his breath. Jim started to pace, feeling tense and worried, and his chest felt even tighter. Soon the tightness began to feel more like an ache and evolved into pain. He asked his brother to call an ambulance. Jim told his doctor later that he thought, "This is it! I'm going to die."

This sort of attention to symptoms is highly selective. That is, you notice and focus on symptoms that you suspect indicate that something is wrong, and you ignore symptoms or sensations that contradict your suspicion. This selectivity is a general principle of psychology: once we think we have an explanation for something—once we've made up our minds—then we only look for information that confirms and supports our explanation, and we ignore information that contradicts it. So if you are worried about the fact that you get dizzy when you stand up suddenly, you notice every time this happens, but you do not notice the times that you stand up and do *not* feel dizzy.

The selectivity of attention makes sense. Your brain is flooded with sensations all the time, and you can only focus your conscious attention on a tiny fraction of them all. If you stop to think about it, you might note that your shoe is too tight, the chair you're sitting in is uncomfortable, or your glasses feel awfully heavy on the bridge of your nose. But we don't usually pay attention to these sensations—they're mild, and they don't suggest that we might be sick, so they don't seem to be worth focusing on. But once you think a sensation might indicate something is seriously wrong, you hone in on it; you scrutinize your body and become hypervigilant. And this only intensifies the sensation.

Attention amplifies bodily symptoms in a number of ways. First, as we've just seen, the more you concentrate on a symptom, the more intense it becomes. Second, because paying attention is such a selective process, it causes you to scan your body for other mild or ambiguous sensations that you hadn't noticed before you became so aware. And there are certainly plenty of mildly uncomfortable sensations around for you to heed. Third, as the symptom intensifies, you become more and more anxious about what it might mean, and the anxiety itself creates additional distressing physical symptoms.

For Jim Reyering and his chest pain, symptom amplification led to a visit to an emergency room.

Doctors ran an electrocardiogram and did a complete physical exam. All the results were normal. Jim couldn't figure out why the pain was not a heart attack until the cardiologist asked him if he had recently overexerted himself. Jim told the doctor about moving the bureau, and the cardiologist explained that Jim's symptoms must have originated with pulling the chest muscles. The cardiologist said he was glad Jim had come in to get evaluated, and that his heart looked very healthy on all counts.

Jim felt reassured when he went home with a clean bill of health. Over the next few weeks, however, he found himself becoming worried again. Every time he drove to work, he passed a billboard advertising the new cardiology hospital in the city. This billboard happened to be on a stretch of road with bad traffic, and Jim was often stressed about being late when he passed the sign. On the billboard was a picture of a man on the golf green clutching at his chest. In huge letters, the sign read, "Is your heart up to par?" After he noticed the billboard, it seemed to Jim that he felt a suspicious tightness in his chest.

At work, Jim received a notice that his life insurance company would require a heart screening from him. He felt the twinge again and began checking himself to see if he could detect any palpitations or numbness. He noticed when he was a little short of breath, and even when he had just come up the stairs he wondered if his heart might be acting up. Sometimes it almost seemed as if he were smothering and couldn't take a deep enough breath.

On his equally stressful drive home from work, a radio ad trumpeted the beneficial effects of aspirin in preventing heart attacks. At the mention of heart attacks, Jim checked for any pain and then took his pulse. Was that a skipped beat?

Jim had passed the billboard every day for a year, and he'd heard that same story on the radio numerous times. But he'd never really thought about them before his father's heart attack. Afterward, every time he saw the billboard or heard the advertisement, his attention went to his heart, his breathing, and his health.

If concentrating on a symptom increases sensitivity and discomfort, it follows that lessening the attention you pay it will decrease discomfort. At the conclusion of a great movie, you may realize you haven't even noticed that chronic heartburn of yours since you first sat down. Very good hypnotic subjects—experts at focusing somewhere other than on symptoms and body sensations—can pay such close attention to the hypnotist's voice and suggestions that they can block out any other incoming sensations. This makes it possible to even perform surgery on such people without using anesthesia, and several burn units in large hospitals use hypnosis to help burn victims with their pain.

In another example of how distraction eases pain, hospital nurses need to give out fewer painkillers to patients during the day than during evening hours. This is because during the day, activities keep the patients busy and visitors distract them, so their pain is less. In the evening, patients are alone and not busy and pay more attention to their pain. Through these examples and studies, we learned that you have the power to improve symptoms by distracting yourself and learning to ignore them.

Distraction is an effective technique for shifting attention away from unpleasant physical sensations or worrisome thoughts. You can distract yourself with hobbies, crafts, household tasks, exercise, music, and countless other activities. Try to focus on a background sound in the room you are in right now. After you've concentrated on that sound for a while, select a sound coming from outside the room and focus on it for a few moments. Once you've gotten good at this, try switching back and forth between the two. You'll notice that this exercise can strengthen your ability to select what you pay attention to.

What have you tried that helped shift attention away from your symptoms? You may do it without even realizing you're using distraction skills. Some patients say they notice symptoms much less while involved in a favorite project or while they are at work. The distraction worksheet at the end of the chapter will give you some more ideas to try.

Relaxation Training

People with distressing and worrisome symptoms become exquisitely sensitive perceivers of bodily sensations. This same sensitivity can be used to your advantage by learning to pay attention to healthy and pleasant bodily sensations instead of distressing and uncomfortable symptoms. With many physical states, such as muscle tension and heart rate, you have the innate ability to make the sensation better. You can capitalize on your sensitivity to become an expert at relaxation.

Relaxation training is proven to be an effective method of reducing stress. Stress in itself causes symptoms because it increases your level of physiological arousal. It increases your heart rate, raises your blood pressure, and causes tensing up of your muscles. Relaxing and calming your mind reverses these stressful changes.

Just as muscle tension and high blood pressure are natural reactions to stress, relaxation is an innate ability that is easy to learn with practice.

Various techniques are used to produce relaxation, including progressive muscle relaxation, a particular form of abdominal breathing, imagery, meditation, prayer, mindfulness, yoga, and tai chi. All meditative techniques have two basic components in common: you learn to focus your attention on a word, phrase, body sensation, or muscular activity; and you take a passive attitude to distracting thoughts when they occur. The second part is the trickiest for many people and causes some to give up on meditation in the first few minutes. It is important to remember that everyone will be distracted by other thoughts (such as laundry that needs to be done, the workday ahead, or your child's dental bills) when trying to focus, especially at the beginning. The key is not to feel guilty for messing up but to gently nudge the thoughts away and focus again, as many times as it takes. In fact, that process of refocusing again *is* the process of meditation and relaxation. Being distracted and then bringing yourself back is all there is to it.

Which relaxation method is best for you depends upon your individual style. Some people experience stress in their bodies as pain or muscle tension. Progressive muscle relaxation (described in the exercises section), yoga, and tai chi are most effective for body tension. Others feel stress in their minds as excessive worry or difficulty concentrating, in which case a mind-focusing approach such as imagery or meditation can be useful. Others find that slow, deep, diaphragmatic breathing is the most relaxing element. Most people feel a combination of mind and body stress; therefore, a combination of techniques is helpful.

Mastering the relaxation response can do more

than help manage chronic symptoms. If practiced regularly, it can reduce anxiety, fear, and panic. It can decrease chronic tension, decrease the risk of heart disease, boost immune function, and improve insomnia. Many of the exercises can be done almost anywhere and at any time. A number of relaxation exercises are fully described and included at the end of the chapter.

We'll return to our example to show how Jim Reyering learned to use relaxation to help his fear and anxiety about his chest pain.

Jim Reyering visited his primary care physician, who had access to Jim's emergency room records. He reassured Jim that his heart was fine and recommended some relaxation techniques to help with stress and anxiety. Jim picked up a book on relaxation from a local bookstore and practiced some of the exercises. The introduction to the book likened relaxation to a "weapon against stress" and emphasized the need for daily practice of the techniques in order for them to be useful in a stressful situation. After all, if Jim were going to use a bow and arrow against an attacking cougar, he had better have a lot of experience with the bow and arrow on a practice field before meeting up with the cougar! The same was true of anxiety and stress. Jim learned to be expert at breathing and letting go of tension while at home in a quiet room. After that, he tried some breathing techniques from the relaxation book while stuck in a traffic jam. He realized that he could ease his palpitations, shortness of breath, and worry with deep breathing and meditation. Instead of his symptoms having control over his life, he used his mind to control his experience of his symptoms.

Exercises

Read through all the exercises first and pick one or two to start. You may not feel that every exercise would be useful for your particular situation, and that's perfectly fine. A good way to continue to practice is to go through the program in the book more than once, and in subsequent readings you may add exercises you didn't do the first time. If you keep each of the exercises you attempt in a single notebook or folder, you can easily follow your progress.

The worksheets and charts work best if they are done daily for the full week. They are designed to help you learn about and track your symptoms from multiple perspectives. The more data you collect, the more you will be able to use this book to effect a change in your life for the better. Once you go on to the next chapter, there is no need to continue the exercises from this chapter unless the exercise says explicitly to continue the practice for more than one week.

PRACTICING ATTENTION AND DISTRACTION

1. Be aware of sensations going on in your body.

Use the first page of your new workbook to simply keep track of sensations in your body for a few hours, or even the whole day. You will be amazed at how many (normal) twinges, itches, gurgles, and pains float through your body all the time—a moment of nausea, a ringing in your ears, a bad taste in your mouth, light-headedness, and belches.

Now look at the list with a new perspective—this list is your reservoir of sensations that you could focus on and misidentify as symptoms of a disease if you were to become worried about being sick. Normally, you'd just dismiss them for what they are, but if you believe them to be connected to some kind of disease, your concern will intensify. How many of these sensations do you spend time worrying about due to a fear of a medical condition, or due to a medical condition you have been diagnosed with and you think is getting worse? The symptoms that really bother you, such as the twinge in Jim Reyering's chest and his shortness of breath, are the ones that we will work on in this six-week program.

2. Track your focus on symptoms.

Write down the symptom that bothers you the most and that has already been checked out by your doctor. Carry an index card around with you for a day and make a note every time you think about the symptom. Are you surprised by how much time you spend thinking about your discomfort, fatigue, or pain? Were there times in the day when you did not think of the symptom? What were you doing during those times? What did you do that made you think about the symptom more? Is there a way to increase the amount of time spent in activities that help you decrease the discomfort from your symptom? Is there a way to minimize or limit the situations, encounters, or activities that make you more aware of the symptom?

3. Learn distraction techniques.

Rate your symptom on a scale of one to five, with five being most bothersome. For five minutes, focus intently on the symptom, thinking about the cause and trying to imagine what is going on inside your body to cause it. Then rate the symptom from one to five again. Which direction did your rating go? Next, select a distraction technique from the following list and practice it for a few minutes. If you want to choose a technique of your own, feel free to do so—any constructive, absorbing activity is a good choice. Distraction can redirect conscious awareness away from bothersome sensations and repeated worries. Rate your symptom again after trying distraction. Did your ratings change? A sample worksheet follows the list of distractions to give you an idea of how to track your responses. Make your own chart similar to our example in your workbook. Complete a row of the worksheet at least once a day for this week.

List of Distractions

- Go through the alphabet, naming varieties of soup. I.e., A=asparagus, B=bean, C=cream of mushroom. Name all the fifty states. Try recalling the names of all your high school or grade school classmates.

- Do a simple task, such as washing dishes, watering plants, fixing something. Give the activity your full attention.

- Spend time on an enjoyable craft project: knitting, needlepoint, woodworking, or stringing beads. Write in a journal, draw, doodle, or paint.

- Focus on the outside world. Stand by the window and count the cars going by. Describe the changes you notice in your garden or front yard since last week.

- Replay a happy moment in your memory as if watching a movie. Use all your senses to make the scene come alive—try to imagine the temperature, the sounds around you, the quality of the light, a breeze, and so on.

- Use rhythm. Sing along with the radio (this works well in the car during a stressful traffic jam), drum with your fingers, recite poetry, or pet a cat.

- Concentrate on planning an activity you are looking forward to.

- Games are a great distraction: try computer games, cards, crossword puzzles, and word games.

- Telephone someone who has a good sense of humor. Deliberately avoid talking about symptoms or health.

- Take a warm bath or shower. Focus on the scent of the soap, the comfort of a fluffy towel. Make it a pleasurable experience.

- Exercise or take a walk.

- Massage your hands/face/neck/shoulders/feet with fragrant lotion.

Jim's Workbook—Attention Exercise Three

Date	Time	Symptom, rating at beginning	Rating after concentrating on symptom for five minutes	Distraction	Effect/ rating after distraction
Jan. 17	10 a.m.	Palpitations barely there... Rating: 1	My heart is going wild. It must be dangerous for it to be racing like this. Rating: 5	Made plans for a camping trip with my brother	Palpitations gone, feeling much more relaxed. Rating: 0
Jan. 18	6 p.m.	Chest tightness— saw that stupid billboard again! Rating: 3	I sat in traffic thinking about my heart...the tightness got worse, of course. Rating: 5	I tried deep breathing for a little while.	The tightness went away, mostly. Rating: 1

Learning Basic Relaxation Exercises

1. THE FUNDAMENTALS OF STRESS-REDUCTION THROUGH MEDITATION AND RELAXATION

Set aside twenty minutes in a quiet room for your first practice. You will find it easier to learn to relax if you do it in the same place every time. Try to reserve that place for your relaxation and meditation exercises; you will find that you will begin to relax simply by sitting down there. Try hanging a "Do Not Disturb" sign on the door so that you and your family will take relaxation seriously. Unplug the telephone. Relaxation should be practiced in a comfortable and supported seating position, not immediately after a meal or when you are hungry. (If you are hungry, have a glass of juice or a piece of fruit before relaxing.) Wear loose clothing. You may find it easiest to concentrate with your eyes closed, but if you prefer your eyes to be open, focus your gaze on an object in front of you or on a spot on the wall.

If you are serious about learning meditation and relaxation as a part of this program, it is important to make the commitment to practice at least five times a week for the first three to four weeks in order to really master the technique and acquire the ability to put yourself in a relaxed state whenever you need to. It is easier to learn to relax if you practice it at the same time each day. This makes it a habit. Do not set a timer. Have a clock available, and when you think the time is up, open your eyes and look. If the time is not up, just close your eyes again and go back to what you were focusing on. If the time is up, close your eyes again and take a moment before slowly opening them again. Taking this moment helps you to carry your relaxed state into your everyday life, instead of suddenly jumping out of meditating or deep breathing just as revved up as you were when you began.

There are normal sensations that accompany relaxation that may feel a bit strange at first. As you become more relaxed, you may notice changes in temperature, your body becoming warmer or cooler. You may notice changes in weight as your arms and legs may feel heavy or light. Muscles may jump or twitch as they do when you are settling down to sleep. Muscles do this naturally when they progress from tension to relaxation and release. All these sensations are positive signals that your relaxation practice is going well. Learning to tolerate these changes and sensations in your body without judgment or fear is part of the reason relaxation is so effective in reducing anxiety and pain from chronic symptoms.

It's important to remember that achieving a truly relaxed state is a skill that you have to learn. Like swimming or riding a bicycle, it takes practice and won't come to you immediately. People often find that they have to practice for several weeks before they start to get the hang of it and feel themselves really able to slip into a truly peaceful, relaxed state. Often, especially at the beginning, your mind will seem even *more* active, and the experience will not be relaxing. That's completely normal—your mind will learn to settle into relaxation and meditation more easily over time.

You may find it's helpful to make a meditation tape, CD, or MP3 playlist. Play a selection of soft music that you like and read the instructions from one of the exercises that follow in a gentle tone over the music. Change your selections as many times as you want, adding exercises or putting in more music without words. If hearing your own voice bothers you, get someone you love to make a tape for you, or purchase one. They are available in almost any store that sells music.

The following exercises begin with the most basic, diaphragmatic breathing, and continue on to cover most of the major forms of relaxation and meditation you can do without extensive demonstration. For tai chi or yoga, it is best to attend a class or purchase a DVD. Begin with diaphragmatic breathing, and then as you become more comfortable, add in the other exercises to the practice. Do your favorite exercise for twenty minutes, or, once you've mastered the basics, choose two or three to do each day. Unlike the other exercises in this chapter, which can be left behind once you complete this week, it is important to continue with meditation, yoga, or another form of relaxation throughout the six weeks. Upcoming chapters will include a few new relaxation exercises to try, but if you find one of these is particularly helpful, you are encouraged to spend at least twenty minutes most days of the next six weeks doing it.

2. DIAPHRAGMATIC BREATHING

One foundation skill of relaxation is diaphragmatic breathing, a particular way of breathing in which you inhale using your diaphragm and your abdomen rather than your chest muscles. Sit comfortably in a chair with both feet flat on the floor. Let your hands rest loosely on your lap or wherever is most comfortable for you. Take a moment to scan your body for any tension. Next, pick a spot on the wall and focus on it while you breathe deeply into your abdomen. Take long, slow, deep breaths, feeling your abdomen move in and out. With exhales, imagine tension flowing out and being released into the air. If your attention drifts from the spot on the wall, gently bring it back into focus. If you become lightheaded or feel dizzy, discontinue the deep breathing and return to your normal breathing rate. If the deep breathing is going well, continue for a few minutes, then move on to Exercise 4 for the remainder of the twenty-minute relaxation session.

3. FURTHER TRAINING IN DIAPHRAGMATIC BREATHING

If you are not sure you are breathing properly in the above exercise, try this sequence. The major breathing muscle of the body is the diaphragm. It is suspended across the bottom of the chest cavity right where your ribs meet your abdomen. The diaphragm moves down during inhalation, and the abdomen expands outward to make room. Deep breathing is facilitated by imagining air flowing into your lungs and down into your abdominal cavity.

Lie on your back, place your hands on your abdomen, and breathe in and out. Notice how the abdomen rises with each inhalation and falls with each exhalation. If you have a hard time noticing this, take your hand and press it into your abdomen as you exhale. When you inhale, your abdomen will push your hand back up.

Next, place one hand on your abdomen and one hand on your upper chest. Take in a deep breath and let it out. With proper diaphragmatic breathing, the hand on the abdomen should move while the hand on the upper chest should hardly move at all. Concentrate on your abdomen moving up and down and the air moving in and out.

You can feel what an abdominal breath is like by exhaling as suddenly and forcefully as you can (pretend you are blowing out a candle) and then immediately interrupt this by breathing in. Because of a neural reflex mechanism, this first inhalation will automatically be a diaphragmatic breath, and that is just the type of breathing that you are trying to learn.

If you still have difficulty with diaphragmatic breathing, try turning so that you lie on your stomach. Rest your head on your hands. Take deep breaths until you can feel your abdomen pushing against and lifting up from the floor. Do this for a few minutes, and then roll over on your back and go to Exercise 4 for the remainder of your twenty-minute relaxation session.

4. ADVANCED DIAPHRAGMATIC BREATHING

Close your eyes or gaze softly at the floor. Take a breath in, and as you exhale, say "ten." Take another breath in a little slower and deeper. As you exhale, say "nine." Continue counting down to zero with each breath. Feel the tension draining out of your body with each exhalation. Repeat this exercise until you have run out of time in your practice session, or until you want to go on to the next relaxation exercise.

5. PROGRESSIVE MUSCLE RELAXATION

Progressive muscle relaxation helps release muscle tension. In this technique you will tense large-muscle groups, focus on the sensation, then release the tension and notice what the muscle feels like when it is truly relaxed. This technique can teach you how to use your muscles to achieve a relaxed state. Start your twenty-minute session with a run-through of the diaphragmatic breathing in Exercise 4, then try the following sequence:

Sit in a comfortable position with your feet flat on the floor. Now flex your right forearm using the bicep muscles in the upper arm. Squeeze tightly and inhale. Count to four, and then exhale as you relax the muscles and release the tension. Notice the difference between loose muscles and tense ones. Some people notice a sensation of warmth or heaviness flowing into the muscle as it is relaxed. Perform the same exercise with your left forearm.

Next, shrug your shoulders up, bringing them as close to your ears as you can. Hold, count to four, then release. Move down to your chest, taking a deep breath, holding, then relax. Pay careful attention to just how the muscles feel when they are fully relaxed. Pull your stomach muscles in and hold tight. Release after counting to four. Next squeeze and release the buttocks, then the muscles of the thighs, and finally the lower legs, counting to four each time. Remember to breathe in with muscle tension and out with relaxation. Notice the difference between loose muscles and tense ones with each muscle group.

Now repeat the exercise in reverse order, starting with the lower legs and moving up, finishing with the arms.

At the end of the exercise, take note of any changes in the tension of your muscles and of any changes in stress or pain in your body.

6. PASSIVE PROGRESSIVE MUSCLE RELAXATION

This is a similar technique to the one taught in the previous exercise, and is often used to decrease stress. Sit in a comfortable position and scan your body for any bits of tension. Let your arms become heavy and relaxed, one at a time. Relax your face, feeling the lines on your forehead become smooth and your jaw loosen. Let your shoulders sag and your neck relax. Continue to breathe deeply as you loosen your back, your seat, and your legs. Let the loose feelings sink down into your calves and feet. Take another deep breath and luxuriate in peace and calm.

7. Learning About Mindfulness

Much of our stress comes from thinking about what has happened and what is going to happen. You become anxious when your thoughts turn to anxiety-provoking subjects, issues that worry, frighten, or frustrate you. If you can develop the skill of deliberately turning your mind away from these thoughts, you will be able to remain in a relaxed frame of mind. Mindfulness is the practice of focusing on the present moment. In this way, worry, anger, and other stressful emotions and thoughts are pushed out of consciousness for the period of meditation, leading to deep relaxation. Try focusing on the mental image of a candle for a minute or two, not letting your attention waver. You can also use a simple phrase or word such as "one" or "peace" or "bread" as a focus point. Try to concentrate for a longer period of time. It is perfectly normal for your thoughts to wander off, perhaps to things that are bothering you or that you are looking forward to, or that you forgot to do earlier in the day. When this happens, just note that your mind has wandered, passively ignore the distracting thoughts, and return to what you were focusing on. Notice how stressed you feel before and after the period of meditation. After some practice with different focus points, try to work on the same focus for five minutes, then ten, then fifteen. Keep doing this exercise up to five times a week, in combination with the previous exercises, so that your total relaxation time is at least twenty minutes a day.

8. Another Mindfulness Exercise— Be Mindful of Sounds

Lie down on your back, resting your hands beside you. Notice the noises around you—cars driving by, the house creaking, an airplane flying overhead, the sound of wind or rain. Now try to listen to these sounds without putting a name to them. Concentrate on the sharpness and pitch of the sound instead. A car going by might make a low rumbling, while its brakes would make a high squealing sound. Being mindful of experiences such as car sounds without automatically jumping to thoughts about cars, traffic, and repair bills can be a useful and relaxing skill. Try this exercise for short periods after starting off with breathing and muscle relaxation. The goal is to observe your sensations and your sensory experience in a neutral, detached fashion. You want to become a disinterested spectator, rather than an interpreter, of what you hear, feel, see, and smell. It is a bit like standing on a bridge, watching the water flow gently past you. You are trying to disengage, to avoid getting caught up in what the sensations mean, what they represent, or what they remind you of.

9. KEEPING A RECORD

Keeping track of your relaxation can help you make sure you are practicing enough, and also help you figure out which techniques work best for you. Here is an example of a relaxation diary:

Date/Time	Exercise	Duration	Comments
May 11, 9 p.m.	Diaphragmatic breathing	Fifteen minutes	Felt more relaxed, worries of the day seemed to lessen.
May 13, 6 a.m.	Meditation	Five minutes	Had a hard time focusing, but it was my first try. Will put on a tape with quiet music next time.
May 14, 6 a.m.	Started with breathing, then moved on to progressive muscle relaxation	Twenty minutes	Wow, I am totally relaxed. I wonder if this feeling will last the rest of the day? Progressive muscle relaxation really seems to work for me.

Brief Relaxation Exercises

Once you have practiced the basic relaxation exercises, try the following brief relaxations. Most of them can be done anytime, anywhere, for a quick calming experience. Good times are when you are put on hold during an important phone call; while sitting in your doctor's waiting room; when someone says something that bothers you; or while standing in line or waiting for the elevator. The more practice you have, the more effective these exercises are during a busy day at work or at a stressful time in your life.

1. Take a stretching break, focusing on tense muscles.

2. Sit in a relaxed position. Ask yourself what muscles you really need to maintain this posture. Relax all the other muscles, letting your body become loose.

3. At work, take a few relaxed breaths, drop your shoulders, and straighten your back. Or pick up a piece of paper and pretend to read it, but actually just focus on one word on the page as you take several relaxed breaths. You can also try standing by a window, daydreaming about being in a special place far away while relaxing your breath and body for a few moments.

4. Sit in a comfortable position, close your eyes, and pay attention to your breathing. Take smooth, deep breaths with your diaphragm. Think about nothing but the air flowing in and out of your body. As you inhale say, "Relax." As you exhale say, "Let go."

5. Count slowly to yourself from ten down to zero, one number for each breath. When you get to zero, see how

you are feeling. If you're feeling better, great! If not, try doing it again.

6. As you inhale, count slowly up to four. As you exhale, count slowly back down to one. Do this several times.

7. In traffic, try this mindful alternative to being annoyed by the antics of drivers around you. Notice your own body sensations instead—the feeling of your foot on the gas and brake pedals, the sensations of acceleration in your body, or the way you feel when noticing flashes of light off of bumpers or the beautiful lines of a car model you admire.

* * *

Now you've learned how attention and focus can cause you to suffer more from the symptoms that you have. We've discussed attention as one of the main influences on how we feel physically, and seen that the amount of attention we pay to symptoms influences how intense these symptoms feel. You've gone through exercises to determine how attention specifically affects your sensations, and have practiced numerous different distraction and relaxation exercises to combat the natural tendency to focus on pain and discomfort.

We cannot stress enough the importance of relaxation exercises, and we will go back to them in future chapters, where you will learn about different aspects of symptom perception and how symptoms affect the way you feel.

CHAPTER FOUR

Week 2—Learn How to Rethink Your Symptoms

This chapter brings together some of the most important concepts in learning to cope with and control medical symptoms. Changing your thinking is key to changing how you feel.

As a living, curious human being, you want to know what is going on and why things happen, both inside yourself and in the world. Your brain combines thoughts, self-talk, assumptions, beliefs, knowledge, and expectations about situations in order to come to conclusions.

What if you heard a loud pop right now? You would naturally wonder whether it was a door slamming, a car backfiring, or maybe even a gunshot. Whenever we first notice something, whether it is a sound or a sensation, our brains will automatically try to explain it. When you notice an uncomfortable bodily sensation, you try to figure out why it is happening, what it might be due to, and what you can do about it. In particular, you almost always wonder what might be causing your symptoms and whether that cause is likely to be benign or something serious. If your hands feel cold as you walk down the street, you might come up with all sorts of reasons about why this is—cold weather, anxiety about a meeting you're about to attend, or even a circulation problem. If you had a medical condition such as diabetes, then a circulation problem could very well exist—but for the most part, worrying about it will not make you feel better, and it certainly won't make your diabetes any better.

Understanding and Misunderstanding the Causes of Symptoms

There is a wide range of benign explanations for symptoms from headaches to fatigue to dizziness to cramps. Overeating, simple "wear and tear," stress, lack of exercise, too little sleep, and normal aging all cause symptoms. These possible explanations normalize the symptom and make it less disturbing. On the other hand, there are also more alarming explanations, such as cancer, a heart attack, or multiple sclerosis. If you have been diagnosed with a disease, you may feel that every time you experience symptoms, they are due to the disease and might indicate that you are getting worse. These are natural thoughts, but they lead to feeling sicker, whether your symptoms are related to your disease or not.

When you believe your symptom is caused by a serious disease or a worsening of your condition, the symptom may become more bothersome, disruptive, and longer-lasting. Sleep apnea is a breathing disorder common to many Americans that can lead to serious health problems. If you have been diagnosed with sleep apnea, worrying about the consequences of the illness heightens your anxiety, making it even harder to fall asleep at night. The longer it takes to fall asleep, the more anxious you get. Thus the worse you think your disorder is, the worse your symptoms become, regardless of whether the disorder itself is worse or not.

Josephine Miller's experience with headaches demonstrates how thinking affects the intensity and anxiety associated with symptoms.

Josephine went to the doctor for severe pain in her jaw. She had started experiencing the pain a few mornings a week, but then it began to happen all the time. She described the pain as being on both sides of her head, near her back molars, and stretching up to her cheeks and down into her neck. Sometimes her jaw was so stiff she could barely move her mouth, and she had begun to sleep with her hand on her cheek, as the warmth seemed to relieve the pain a little bit. The pain had been affecting her sleep, and what finally brought her in to see the doctor was something she read on the Internet. She saw that headaches that awaken people from sleep could be due to brain tumors. Josephine had been diagnosed with a noncancerous brain tumor ten years before, and it had been successfully surgically removed. Every year she had a head scan to make sure her tumor had not come back, and this year's scan had been completely normal. She thought it would be wise to go to the doctor just to make sure it was not her tumor coming back. Her primary care physician noticed that she was exhausted, fearful, and close to tears when talking about her pain.

Her doctor did a thorough neurological exam and found nothing wrong. She then explained to Josephine that daily headaches are usually caused by muscle tension, which can be quite painful but is not deadly. Since Josephine's last head scan had been only a month before the headaches began, and the type of tumor Josephine had ten years ago tends to grow very slowly, the doctor thought it would be extremely unlikely that the tumor had come back. Josephine didn't know whether to believe her or not—muscle tension? That seemed too simple an explanation for her symptoms.

Many medical students fall prey to the powerful way in which thoughts, ideas, and information shape our perceptions of our bodies. When the students begin to treat patients for the first time and learn about diseases they never knew about before, sometimes they start to experience the symptoms of those diseases. Old aches and pains they had previously ignored now have new, ominous explanations and so they become aware of them. Tinnitis, or ringing in the ears, happens to almost everyone, but medical students will often notice it in themselves when they are learning about the rare forms of brain tumors that cause ringing in the ears.

Medical students can be quite inventive about which form of a disease they might have, and these alarming thoughts make the symptoms seem worse. Often, the students end up seeking medical attention. A typical example is a medical student who was assigned a young male patient hospitalized with a rapidly progressing case of multiple sclerosis. As the student read up on multiple sclerosis in the textbook, he learned all of its possible symptoms and that it tends to strike young adults. When he was shaving, he noticed in the mirror that the lower half of his face was not quite symmetrical. Immediately he concluded this was the earliest sign that he had developed multiple sclerosis. The reality is that he had been looking at that same asymmetry in the mirror every morning for years—but he never noticed it because it never had any significance for him until he learned that it could be a symptom of a serious disease.

Patients describe this same type of thinking. After his fiftieth birthday, an insurance agent noticed that he seemed to be feeling more tired than when he was younger, and that he was more breathless after climbing a flight of stairs. But he figured he was just getting out of shape, since he had gradually stopped regular exercise. Then one day, a coworker told him he looked pale. He began to wonder whether he had anemia, since he had heard that anemia makes you look pale. Once that suspicion was planted in his mind, he was on the lookout for other symptoms that would confirm his fears. Now, when he climbed a flight of stairs he decided that that same breathlessness was due to anemia.

Research studies prove that we all can fall prey to this kind of thinking. When a large number of healthy factory workers underwent screening chest X-rays, a few were found to have suspicious results that could possibly be evidence of heart disease. Almost no one turned out to be sick after they were fully evaluated, but 8 percent of the workers developed cardiac symptoms—just from being told they might possibly have something wrong with their hearts.[1]

The nightly news, magazines, and newspapers are a common source of new and often disturbing information. Every week we hear about dreadful new diseases— SARS, "flesh-eating bacteria," West Nile virus, anthrax, Ebola, mad cow disease, deadly *E. coli* in hamburgers, Lyme disease, and so on. Sometimes just hearing about the disease plants a seed of suspicion about a longstanding, familiar sensation, and we scan our bodies for the other symptoms mentioned in the story. Here is an example of how easy it is to worry about the overload of negative information we learn every day:

I got several mosquito bites last week while working in the yard. And I've had night sweats for the last two nights. Maybe I've developed a fever. Could it be the beginning of West Nile virus or Lyme disease? The more I focus on the feeling of being hot and sick, the more my cheeks feel flushed and the weaker I feel. I hope I'm not really sick.

When a celebrity gets sick and the news is broadcast on TV or written about in newspapers, people wonder if they might have the same disease. At that point they notice mild symptoms that have been there for a long time but which were mostly ignored before. If you're thinking about a heart attack, gas pain feels a lot like chest pain; after you've read about President Reagan's Alzheimer's disease and you forget a phone number, you wonder if your memory might be starting to fail. In Boston, after basketball star Reggie Lewis died suddenly of an irregular heartbeat on the court, many frightened young men who had had palpitations for years but had ignored them as insignificant now came to cardiac clinics asking for an electrocardiogram. Like most healthy people, they had never paid any attention to these occasional skipped beats until they heard about this new, worrisome, possible cause for them.

The same sort of thing happens to people who have had a cancer treatment. Since they fear a return of the cancer, every innocent joint ache or pain in an extremity could signal that the cancer has recurred. This is a perfectly normal and understandable reaction. But the point is that our ideas and our suspicions about these benign aches and pains can make them much worse.

People often have beliefs that make it harder for them to be reassured that their condition is not dangerous or harmful. For example, many patients believe that if they are not having their symptoms at the moment when a medical test is performed, a normal test result is false and can't be trusted. Others believe that serious disease can only be truly ruled out with laboratory tests, so if their physician attempts to reassure them without having performed any tests, this reassurance falls on deaf ears. For those who are ill with diseases such as psoriasis, emphysema, or hepatitis C, the problem is the same. A normal liver-function test may not reassure you that your hepatitis is not getting any worse. For those with and without diagnosed diseases, thoughts and beliefs about your symptoms and whether they mean that your illness is getting worse influence how bad you feel.

Confirmatory Bias, Anticipation, and Future Expectations

Besides influencing current symptoms, your ideas about your present state of health have a big influence on your future symptoms. It is the power of suggestion: beliefs shape future perceptions by creating expectations about what you will experience next. Josephine Miller knew she was going to wake up with a headache every morning, so every night she went to bed more tense than she did the night before. That led to her tension headaches getting worse and worse.

Once you think you have an explanation for a perception, you will selectively search for further information to substantiate the suspicion. Evidence that fails to confirm your suspicion will be ignored. For example, if you are worried that you get sinus troubles from the air quality in the building where you work, you take special note of the times you have a stuffy nose at work. You may not notice all the days you go to work and breathe just fine.

Imagine you are walking through the forest and out of the corner of your eye you see a thin, curvy brown form on the ground. You might assume that it is a snake. If you then hear a rustling sound, you will conclude that this is the sound of the snake rustling around. Having come to this conclusion, you don't make any attempts to find alternative explanations for the sound, so you don't look up to see that there is a breeze rustling the leaves. By focusing on the assumption that the form you noticed was a snake, you prevent yourself from noticing other evidence that could change your mind and help you discover a less alarming explanation for the sound.

The same kind of thinking naturally leads to fear and anxiety about symptoms. Unfortunately, fear and anxiety only make your symptoms worse. Anxiety over a serious disease can lead to illogical thinking. For example, "Multiple sclerosis can cause tingling sensations; therefore, because I've developed tingling, I must have MS." While not as humorous as Woody Allen's famous example of faulty logic—"Socrates is a man; all men are mortal; therefore, I am Socrates"—this sort of temporary lapse in our powers of rational thinking is very common when we become alarmed. The answer is to consider other possible causes for symptoms—to learn how to seek reassurance rather than look for more reasons to be distressed. This may seem too straightforward, too simple, to work. But medical research has proven that the simple act of changing your thoughts can change your symptoms, and improve your life.

Developing Alternative Explanations

How do you change your beliefs about the causes and progression of symptoms? A good way to start, whether you have been diagnosed with a disease or not, is by developing a better appreciation of the ordinary, nondisease-related causes of symptoms. We're used to seeing health as the glowing examples of movie stars and fitness models. But in the real world, the state of normal health is often accompanied by a variety of benign discomforts and illnesses that last for a short while or come and go. As Lewis Thomas has noted, "The great secret...is that most things get better by themselves. Most things, in fact, are better by morning."[2] Headaches and backaches, stiffness, rashes, ringing in the ears, upper respiratory symptoms, and diarrhea are commonplace in perfectly healthy people. Surveys indicate that 86–95 percent of the general public experiences at least one such symptom in a given two- to four-week interval, and the typical adult has at least one symptom every four to six days. Thus painful, recurrent sore throats are most often nothing more than that— recurrent sore throats—and not due to leukemia or some rare immune deficiency. This doesn't mean that they aren't bothersome and disruptive, but it does mean that you needn't compound the pain with the worry that the pain could mean something far worse. To take another example, nosebleeds *can* indicate high blood pressure—but far more often they are merely nosebleeds.

The ability to consider alternative, more benign explanations for a symptom, rather than jumping to the conclusion that it is caused by a worsening of your condition or by a new disease, will help you reassure yourself and keep the symptom in perspective. The vast majority of unpleasant sensations originate from normal causes. Increased muscle tension can cause headaches, fatigue, weakness, and aching. Rapid, shallow breathing can cause dizziness, faintness, numbness, and tingling. Overexertion can cause muscle and joint pain and fatigue. Lack of sleep leads to muscle soreness, general malaise, and memory and concentration problems. Dietary indiscretion can cause burning, bloating, and pain. Caffeine causes palpitations. Emotional upset or anxiety can cause a rapid heartbeat, sweating, shortness of breath, trouble concentrating, and nausea.

Having appreciated this perspective, you can now consider alternative explanations for your symptoms. Why is this helpful? Because alternative explanations can reduce the heart-stopping fear that comes from thinking about a deadly cause for symptoms. Remember, the chances of having a deadly symptom compared to a benign one are miniscule. Those with diagnosed diseases get plenty of benign symptoms too. Human brains seem to be hard-wired to exaggerate the chances of having a serious disease and distort the likelihood of something terrible happening. We anticipate not the most *likely* thing but the most *catastrophic* thing. If you don't want to live with so much fear and distress, try to change your beliefs by changing how you think and talk to yourself. Changing your beliefs about a symptom can change how the symptom feels.

Could it really be that easy? Take a minute right now to think about headaches. Imagine a throbbing ache in the middle of your forehead. Think of bright lights and loud music and babies crying. Do you start to feel the ache? Does it get worse when you think about a freight train chugging away in your head, or a deadline at work, or a sick relative? Many people will get a mild headache while reading this paragraph. That's how powerful the mind is in controlling symptoms. If you still feel the headache, rub your forehead and take a few deep breaths. Imagine a quiet, dark place. Symptoms, whether they are from a diagnosable disease or not, can be made worse through maladaptive thoughts. Fortunately, the reverse is also true. Symptoms can be made better through the constructive thoughts you are learning and practicing in this book.

Josephine Miller talked with her doctor about the timing of her tension headaches. Her doctor thought it was pretty telling that Josephine's headaches began to get a lot worse after Josephine started to worry about her brain tumor coming back. Josephine realized that her worry about the brain tumor caused tremendous anxiety and her headaches got a lot worse with the added worry.

But how could anxiety cause so much pain? The intensity of the pain seemed to confirm her concern that she had something horrible like a brain tumor. Josephine was skeptical that something as simple as anxiety could cause such intense physical symptoms. Then her doctor asked her if she had ever felt any of the same kind of pain in her life. Josephine remembered that when she was a teenager, on the mornings of tryouts for band and orchestra, she would wake up with splitting headaches. Of course, back then, she didn't worry about brain tumors. She realized that the explanation was anxiety about the music competition.

It hardly seems fair that our body experiences so many things as painful and distressing. However, these benign sensations can be dealt with by recognizing the connection between the symptom and the cause and trying a commonsense or self-care intervention. For example, when you notice that your breathing is rapid and shallow, slow down and substitute the diaphragmatic breathing learned in the previous chapter.

Cognitive Restructuring

You have now learned in detail how the way we think affects the way we feel, and you were introduced to the concept of developing alternative explanations. That ability is only one piece of a powerful tool known as cognitive restructuring. We've been using our brain to think our whole lives, and we all develop habitual thinking patterns. These patterns are so automatic that we hardly notice them, yet they make up our worldview and limit our ability to create new ways to cope with old problems. So far we've focused on how believing our symptoms are caused by a serious or worsening medical condition can make us feel worse; now we will talk about negative thinking in general, what it does to your symptoms, and how to change it.

Take some time today to notice your thoughts about your family and friends, what you see around you, and what you hear. If you've never paid attention to this before, you'll be surprised—every day we have a running dialogue in our heads, criticizing, advising, wishing, anticipating, and explaining.

"My head is going to explode," thought Joesphine one morning before going into work. "I can't handle this pain! It's never going to end! But if I were tough enough, I would be able to handle it."

Josephine, in her pain, tortured herself with her own thoughts. If you have a chronic medical symptom, chances are you spend a lot of time thinking about your condition. And your usual ways of thinking *are* affecting the pain or discomfort you feel. But what if you could change the way you think, and therefore change the way you feel?

The technique of cognitive restructuring is a valuable tool for managing medical symptoms. Cognitive restructuring is the process of replacing the old, habitual negative thoughts that lead to feeling distress into new more hopeful thoughts that enhance the ability to cope.

Here are the five basic steps of cognitive restructuring:

1. Take notice of what you are thinking, and track negative automatic thoughts. How and when do you talk to yourself about a symptom? These thoughts might be short phrases, or even visual images. Perhaps they lead to feeling anxious or upset. Think about the steps you take from first noticing the sensation to when you start to feel

worse. Your first thought when you feel a symptom may also be something negative about the symptom itself— "That chest pain will never get better"; "It will keep me from doing things I really want to"; "It's going to end up shortening my life"; or "Maybe it's an inherited condition and my kids will get it."

2. Recognize the responses, both physical and nonphysical, that follow the thought. Does the thought make you feel nervous or irritable? Does it make your preexisting symptoms worse? Does your heart rate speed up, or your breathing get shallow? How do your muscles feel, loose or tense?

3. Develop rational countering statements for each thought, based on realistic alternative explanations.

4. Replace the negative automatic thought with a rational statement that puts the symptom in perspective and helps you feel more in control. Notice the change in the emotional and physical responses when you use the countering thought. You will notice a change in your negative feelings and anxiety levels if you think, for example, "Though my arthritis does flare up and get worse at times, it always calms down again afterward," or "I've dealt with this before, and I can do it again."

5. Practice! Each time you catch yourself focusing attention on a familiar, benign symptom, notice the thoughts and then challenge any distressing beliefs with alternative explanations and reassuring statements. Just as we build strong muscles by repeated exercising, we build healthy thoughts by repeating rational thoughts. The thoughts we repeat most become the strongest. Every motivational speaker and guru knows this and makes it the cornerstone of his or her program for success.

Cognitive restructuring is one of the most powerful tools used in this book, but it does take practice. After all, you may have been repeating negative thoughts for years, until they have become unconscious habits—automatic reflexes. With enough skill, this technique can change the way the outside world affects you. You have more control over what you think and feel in a positive way. The exercises at the end of this chapter will illustrate this technique and help make cognitive restructuring second nature to you.

One young man noticed that his nausea and indigestion seemed worse when he was in a room full of people. The nausea was so bad it kept him from the gym, and working out had been one of his favorite activities. After learning about cognitive restructuring, he traced his thought patterns from the moment he entered into a social situation. His first thought was, *They're not going to like me.* Every interaction he had from that point on was colored by his negative thoughts; he became nervous and wasn't up to the task of talking to others. His anxiety made his stomach feel worse. It was hard enough just to be in the room, but then he started worrying that he might even throw up. Of course, no one would come up to him to talk, since he appeared uncomfortable and anxious. And people's avoidance of him just seemed to prove his point. He was so used to thinking negatively that he didn't notice it until he stopped to observe himself.

The next time he entered a room with a lot of people, he automatically thought, *They're not going to like me.* But this time he was ready. He knew there was no reason to think this. In social situations involving a small group of friends, when he wasn't nauseated, everyone liked him just fine, and enjoyed conversing with him. He countered his initial, negative thought with, *There is no reason not to like me.* It worked—he smiled, because the familiar symptoms didn't start. People joined in conversations with him, and he actually began to enjoy himself.

His indigestion didn't go away immediately. Sometimes he forgot to notice his thoughts, and the old negative ones came back. But as he practiced more in those social situations that he had avoided, he got better and better at stopping his automatic thoughts before they led to discomfort and anxiety.

Once we've learned how to notice and take control over our own inner voices, we can see how this inner dialogue combines with certain circumstances and situations to make symptoms continue or get worse. We'll explore more about the specifics of situations in the next chapter.

Josephine Miller learned to recognize her negative thoughts when they happened. Instead of dwelling on what she couldn't handle, she decided to do things that could help her cope. She learned to counter the thought "If I were tough enough, I would be able to handle it" with the thought "I've been able to overcome other problems in the past, so I'll be able to cope with this one too." She used some meditation exercises every night before she went to bed, and noticed she woke up less anxious and with less pain than she had in the past. Since her headaches had started to abate, she decided that they couldn't be due to a brain tumor and now ascribed them to work-related stress. By figuring out how negative thinking affected her physical sensations, she was able to stop making herself worse and start focusing on ways to decrease her headaches naturally, without pain medicine, and without side effects.

The exercises and worksheets in this chapter are meant to help you figure out how your thinking is related to your symptoms. The more you train your mind to think in different ways about your symptoms, the less you will be stuck in the same old patterns of pain and distress.

Exercises

1. Recognize your negative thoughts.

What immediately comes to mind when you think about the possible causes of your symptom? Do you have an ominous explanation, as Josephine Miller did? Your first task is to monitor and identify the alarming cognitive distortions and worrisome images that your symptoms trigger. Take note of your negative thoughts for the next couple of hours as you go through the normal routine of your day. It's helpful to carry a notebook with you to jot down your thoughts as they occur. How do those negative thoughts make you feel? Are they helpful in any way? Are they harmful?

Josephine's Workbook for Exercise One

Recognizing negative thoughts—here are some I noticed myself thinking today:

"Because my headaches are so severe, they must be caused by my brain tumor coming back."

"I can't take it anymore! How could anyone put up with this?"

"Plenty of people go to work with a lot more serious problems than a stupid headache. I must be weak."

Wow—I never noticed before just how negative I am. Just reading over these thoughts makes me feel bad. I'm just spending time waiting for my headache to come back. How could these thoughts be helpful? As they are, I don't see any way. Maybe if I were less critical, for example, stopping my third thought with "Plenty of people have more serious problems," and not going forward with "I must be weak," then I might have some perspective on my headaches without beating myself up about them.

2. Learn to develop alternative explanations.

You've already begun the process of listing negative thoughts when they happen, and you realize just how much they contribute to feeling worse. The next step in cognitive restructuring is to develop alternative explanations for your negative thoughts. For each thought you wrote down in Exercise 1, answer the following questions:

- Does this thought contribute to my symptoms?
- Where did I learn this thought?
- Is it a logical thought?
- Is the thought actually true?

Now try to develop an alternative explanation for your symptoms, following Josephine's example:

Alternative explanation for headache—muscle tension, caused by stress.

- *Once in a while, especially on the weekends, I wake up without any headache.*
- *My headaches were much worse the week we started that tough project at work.*
- *Deep breathing and relaxation improve the soreness around my neck and jaw.*
- *My doctor told me my neurological examination was normal.*
- *Anxiety, stress, and muscle tension are much more common than brain tumors.*

3. Create a worksheet to track your negative thinking over time.

Keeping a record of your thoughts for a week can be very revealing. You might be surprised about how negative your thoughts are or how much you think about your symptoms. The more you know about your mind-body connection, the more you can use it to feel better. Each time you have a symptom over the course of the next week, record it in the symptoms column of your worksheet. In the First Thoughts column, record the initial thoughts that arise when each symptom begins. In the Alternative Explanation column, record a more healthy alternative thought.

Symptoms and Thoughts Worksheet

Date	Time	Symptom	First Thoughts	Alternative Explanation
Jan. 17	8 a.m.	Headache	I'm waking up with the headache again—what if it is a brain tumor?!	Headaches can be caused by muscle tension and anxiety. I'm nervous about the staff meeting... there may be more layoffs.
Jan. 19	8:45 a.m.	Headache	This is so horrible—how am I going to face that meeting today?	I've run this meeting a hundred times—I'll be able to run it today, too.

4. Practice positive talk.

Write down ten positive things about yourself. Say them aloud. Do you feel better, or just silly? How would you speak to a friend with similar problems to yours? Would you be harsh and condemning, or compassionate? Just as it does not help to be cruel to a friend who is in a tough situation, it is rarely a good idea to be cruel to yourself. Kindness and reinforcement is a much more effective way to support yourself though difficult times and painful symptoms. Keep saying positive things about yourself until you get a sense of positive reinforcement.

5. Track your thoughts daily, and take your practice cards with you.

If a symptom is bothering you so much that it intrudes on your daily life and work, write a negative automatic thought about the sensation on one side of an index card. On the other side write an alternative explanation. There is an example below, and you can use a thought and alternative explanation from the previous exercise. Keep the card with you and use it whenever you experience the negative thought. The repetition will help undo the automatic negative thought and replace it with an automatic alternative explanation. Remember, we believe what we tell ourselves, so make your thoughts contribute to feeling better!

Josephine's Index Cards

front

I'm so tired—there must be something seriously wrong with me.

back

These headaches are interfering with my sleep. That will make me tired. It's not my tumor coming back—that never made me tired.

front

I can't handle these headaches one more minute!

back

Of course I can. I've dealt with them so far, and now I'm working in positive ways to cope with them.

6. Continue to use relaxation techniques.

This week, try to set aside twenty minutes on at least five days for your relaxation practice. Continue using the techniques and log you began in Chapter 4.

*   *   *

The ways in which we think, talk to ourselves, and decide what to believe have a powerful impact on symptoms. There are ways of thinking that make symptoms feel worse, and ways of thinking that make symptoms feel better. Thinking styles can influence current sensations and perceptions, and create expectations about future experiences. When we pick up new information, it can lead to reinterpreting old symptoms as new and serious diseases.

Just as Josephine developed alternative explanations and found ways to combat the real culprit behind her headaches—stress and negative thinking—we hope you have used the techniques in this chapter to learn a great deal more about how you think about your symptoms. This knowledge will not only help undo the effects of negative thinking, but will protect you in the future by helping you recognize when negative automatic thoughts affect how you feel.

CHAPTER FIVE

Week 3—Change the Situation, Lessen Your Symptom

You've heard the expression "Beauty is in the eye of the beholder." Well, so is bodily distress. How bad something hurts, how bothersome a symptom is, depends in large measure on how you view it, what your vantage point on it is, what context you put it in. Those new contact lenses feel very uncomfortable at the beginning until you're reassured that the sensation is temporary and perfectly normal. Sweetbreads may taste great until you learn what they are. The intensity of many different sensations depends on your perspective. A young couple sneaking home down a dark street perceives the corner streetlight to be glaringly bright. The worried parents, waiting on the porch, perceive that same light to be too dim.[1]

You may have noticed that your thoughts are more upsetting and your symptoms are especially bothersome in particular situations. Banging your shin on the table on your way to the bathroom in the middle of the night probably hurts a lot more than the same injury in the middle of your annual Superbowl party, when you are distracted by your friends and the game. How we experience our symptoms depends on the context and circumstances we are in at the time. If you've been hearing a lot recently about "cancer clusters" or "toxic buildings," and then a coworker is diagnosed with leukemia, you may fixate on the fact that you've lost a pound or two, or that you seem to bruise awfully easily.

The common feature of these situational factors is that they tend to direct attention to our bodies; they make us doubt our health and interpret bodily discomfort as more serious and ominous. As we have seen, these factors may amplify the original symptom. A key skill in managing medical symptoms is figuring out which conditions make your symptoms worse, and then changing those conditions as much as possible.

"I'm so tired all the time," Caroline says to herself as she climbs the short flight of stairs to the entrance of the medical building. It used to be that her daughter would take Caroline to her arthritis appointments, but her daughter moved away about three months ago. Now each day seems to take extra effort. Why does her doctor's office have to be up a flight of stairs? Her fatigue, along with the aching in her joints, leaves her feeling exhausted. "I'm just not strong enough anymore to do much of anything."

Caroline's visit to her doctor is not reassuring. The doctor, running late, impatiently asks about Caroline's sleep, appetite, and mood, but seems to dismiss her complaint of fatigue. Though Caroline admits to feeling a little down about her daughter's move and is having trouble with her sleep, she doesn't see how her overwhelming lack of energy could be connected to the doctor's questions. She's heard of people with cancer or chronic viruses who go for months with symptoms of fatigue without being diagnosed properly. Caroline is incensed when her doctor gives her a referral to a psychiatrist. Out of politeness, she takes the appointment slip, but she leaves the doctor's office so furious that she is clenching her fists. Now her hands ache, she's more exhausted than ever, and her doctor thinks she is crazy!

Circumstances that often affect symptoms include stressful events, interpersonal relationships, timing, expectations, conditioned habits, and the limitations of medical knowledge and treatment. Can you think of some people or personal habits that make your symptom feel better or worse? Like a journalist, you can use the "five Ws"—who, what, why, when, and where—to investigate all aspects your specific situation.

Let's consider the context when Caroline was really bothered by her fatigue. She was at the doctor's office, having a checkup with a hurried doctor. She's in an unfriendly medical building and feels misunderstood about her symptoms. She's stressed, anxious, and angry in a place where the main focus is health and symptoms. No wonder she feels even more worn out.

When a new symptom develops, it is natural to look to current circumstances for clues about what the sensation means and how important it is. If you sneeze when someone else in the family has a cold, you might initially think that you have caught the cold, even without any other symptoms. What if your family was healthy, your wife had just shaken out a rug, and you sneezed? You might attribute the sneeze to dust in the air, and not think any more about it.

We decide what we ought to be feeling—or not feeling—in light of our current circumstances. Take as an example the phenomenon of "epidemic hysteria" that sometimes happens among groups of adults or children. Epidemic hysteria most commonly occurs in groups of people who are closely confined together or are very familiar with each other, like campers at a summer camp, attendees at a weekend retreat, or coworkers at a stressful job. An outbreak begins when someone is suddenly taken ill. For example, someone in a group may faint, vomit, or have a seizure. A sense of alarm rapidly develops and spreads through the group as the people nearby worry that they might also be overcome by something contagious or toxic that they have all been exposed to. What if there is a gas leak in the ventilation system, or food poisoning from something they've all just eaten?

The people near the affected person begin experiencing alarming symptoms similar to those of the person originally overcome—symptoms such as lightheadedness, dizziness, shortness of breath, or nausea. The outbreak spreads through the group. Eventually, the contagion stops spreading, and in the end, no infectious agent or toxic exposure is ever found to account for people's symptoms. What actually happens in these situations is that the bodily symptoms of anxiety—rapid shallow breathing, racing heart, trembling, dizziness, feeling faint, nausea—are all mistaken as signs of succumbing to the spreading illness, when in fact they are caused by anxiety and stress.

At the opposite extreme is the phenomenon of battlefield anesthesia, in which some soldiers seriously wounded in combat may experience little or even no pain. They request fewer painkillers than civilians with similar injuries sustained in accidents.[2] This difference in the experience of pain is due to the differing contexts: what has happened to the soldier is not unexpected, is happening to others all around him, and at least means that he has not been killed; the civilian's accident, on the other hand, is unanticipated and not congruent with anything happening to others around him.

Caroline tells her daughter about her visit to the doctor. Her daughter moved from the house they shared to a town several hours away and worries about her mother being alone. Her daughter suggests that she see the psychiatrist, so she can talk to someone about coping with her constant fatigue. Caroline is upset at first, but then she realizes that perhaps her daughter has a point. Caroline has stopped taking her morning walks and spends most of her days in front of the television. She knows that without her daughter's help with the mortgage, she will have to move to a condominium. Just the thought of moving all of her possessions overwhelms her.

She has no real interest in anything that's on TV—she just switches channels back and forth. She's even given up knitting, her favorite hobby, because she is just too tired, and even thinking about knitting makes her hands hurt. In fact, looking at her chair by the window with her bag of yarn and needles causes a tired feeling in her back. Her daughter calls, and her first question is about how Caroline feels and how tired she is. Caroline thinks, Why should my illness have to be the most important thing in my life, even affecting my relationship with my daughter? She decides to keep the appointment with the psychiatrist.

Symptoms as an Interpersonal Communication

Interpersonal factors are an important part of your circumstances, and they can have a strong influence on the perception and expression of symptoms. People tend to have habitual ways of making their own needs known and of responding to other people's wishes. Sometimes these communication styles help you handle the situation, but other communication styles can lead to frustration on both sides. When you are communicating about a symptom, the symptom can become better or worse depending on the nature of that communication process.

How do you communicate to your family that you are not feeling well? In answering that question, don't forget about nonverbal communication—such as taking a pill, grimacing, limping, rubbing a part of your body. Do you ask others for help with a chore or simply tell them how poorly you are feeling? How do you think they should respond? Which responses make you feel better? Which responses make your symptoms feel worse or last longer? If you're not sure how your family communicates, imagine a video camera filming your interactions for a day. If an observer watched the tape with the sound off, how would he or she know you were sick?

A striking example of how symptoms can be used as nonverbal communication in families was discovered in a famous study carried out with adolescents who had diabetes.[3] In families where parents were threatening to get divorced, the child's diabetes often got out of control and required hospitalization just when the parents were most at odds and their marriage was at the breaking point. The child had inadvertently discovered that when his or her diabetes required hospitalization, the parents would stop fighting with each other and come together in order to care for their seriously ill child. Thus the child's symptoms had become a way of holding the family together, whereas simply pleading with the parents not to separate had little effect.

Clare Morales told her doctor that her two youngest sons refused to listen to her medical complaints, but her oldest son was very sympathetic. She realized that she only called him when she was very upset or needed a ride to the hospital. Since she craved his company, she noticed her symptoms came on more frequently. She decided to try calling him for discussions about nonmedical topics on a few nights a week and planning a pleasant activity on weekends. With considerable effort, they both felt more relaxed, and her symptoms improved.

Symptoms can become a way of trying to say something to other people with a bodily language rather than with words. Often, when we're feeling in need of assistance or special attention, telling others about a worsening symptom or reminding them of our illness can be a subtle way of asking for their help and special consideration. If we can find a way to ask directly, however, we discover that the symptom doesn't have to be so intense in order to get the help or attention from our families that we seek. Frank Faraar felt funny about asking his wife for a back rub when he wanted one. But he had discovered inadvertently that she would stop paying so much attention to their three children and pay more attention to him, and even give him a back rub, when his lumbago was "acting up again."

Caroline keeps her appointment with the psychiatrist, and he asks a lot of questions about Caroline's situation, especially about the timing of her fatigue and her daughter's move. He asks how she is handling the stress and the bills, living by herself. Caroline admits it has been very difficult—and exhausting. The psychiatrist also reviews Caroline's medical history and her medications, and sends her for some blood tests. Caroline is disappointed in the psychiatrist—he doesn't tell her anything about what might be causing her symptoms. The psychiatrist is just like every other doctor: he listens, says nothing, and sends her for tests.

In the time between psychiatric appointments, Caroline is extremely worried that her blood test results will show something terrible. She spends her days closed up in her house and doesn't call her daughter or her friends. She becomes more exhausted, and her hands become so stiff she can barely move them. Her last unfinished knitting project is still in her craft bag next to her chair. Her daughter is so concerned about not hearing from her that she comes to visit each weekend between appointments.

Future Expectations

Another major factor that you must assess in the circumstances surrounding your symptoms is your expectations about the future. Circumstances and situations tell us what to anticipate will happen next, and future expectations are powerful symptom amplifiers. Waiting expectantly for someone who is late to finally arrive may cause us to hear footsteps down the hall that we would not have heard otherwise. In the same way, expecting to feel sick turns up the volume on any uncomfortable bodily sensation. By figuring out exactly which situations turn up the volume on your symptoms, you can gain perspective on whether the symptom is truly worse, or whether the situation is the real culprit. Have you ever had a cold on a plane? With blocked-up ears, the pain from atmospheric pressure changes on takeoff can be excruciating. The whole plane ride, you imagine the landing and how horrible it will be. Maybe you take a decongestant, but you worry that the trip won't be long enough for it to kick in. Every moment of the descent, you expect the pain to come back, and every small change of pressure or twinge of discomfort in your ear makes you wince in anticipation of more pain.

Future health expectations alter the way we perceive our present health. This often occurs when people in pain believe that relief is imminent. Anticipating that our suffering *should* be going away but *isn't* makes it worse. One man described sitting in the ophthalmologist's waiting room, waiting for his doctor to see him and give him something to ease the pain of a scratch he had just received on his eye. Even though the injury was not getting worse, the pain intensified as the minutes went by, since the anticipated relief was tantalizingly close but had not quite come yet.

Expectations and beliefs about long-standing symptoms can definitely influence our perception of health. Expecting that a symptom will vanish with treatment makes its persistence worse than if you had never expected relief in the first place. It can be very hard to hear that a physician cannot completely cure a symptom, or that a distressing illness just has to run its course. But unfortunately, the truth is that medical science is limited in its ability to treat many of the ailments of daily life and common, benign afflictions. Complete relief is not just around the corner—sometimes we just have to learn how to live better with our symptoms. Living with our symptoms and learning to manage them, rather than engaging in a futile battle to erase them completely, helps us maintain control over how we feel. Part of managing symptoms is recognizing the physical circumstances that worsen them.

Conditioned habits also influence how we experience physical urges. We associate sitting in the kitchen with eating, so sometimes we can bring on the urge to snack just by sitting down in the kitchen, even if we aren't hungry. Smokers who are in the habit of having a cigarette with their morning cup of coffee find there is such a strong connection between the smoking and the coffee that they have to give up coffee while trying to stop smoking. This habituation can also affect symptoms. If you always rest in the same reclining chair when you have pain in your back, you might start to associate that chair with pain. When you walk into the room and see the chair, you may notice that your back hurts even if you weren't aware of the pain a few minutes earlier.

Rick Prentice realized that whenever his boss approached, his stomach gurgled, and the burning sensation of acid reflux worsened. He had become conditioned to associating the boss's presence and his frequent demands for overtime work with his burning and pain. Once he recognized what was amplifying his pain, Rick found it helpful to consciously relax as the boss approached, and he became more assertive about setting limits on overtime. His heartburn improved and no longer came on cue when his boss entered the room. Once you can identify the physical circumstances and interpersonal situations that make symptoms worse, you can work on avoiding or changing them.

Lois Adler became terribly nauseated during the chemotherapy she had to undergo for lymphoma. She noticed she felt ill every time she entered her breakfast room, and then realized that the color of the walls was the same color as the room in which she had her chemotherapy infusions. After she told her husband, he repainted the breakfast room, and her morning nausea went away.

At the long-awaited follow-up appointment, the psychiatrist tells Caroline he doesn't think she is very depressed, but that he worries that she became so tired after her daughter moved away. He shows her the lab results, which are all normal, and emphasizes that no bad news is actually good news. Many very serious conditions, such as kidney disease and leukemia, have been ruled out by the tests. The psychiatrist is concerned that her new habit of staying immobile all day may be contributing to her fatigue and even worsening her arthritis by causing excess stiffness from disuse. He encourages her to take up walking again, with the approval of her arthritis doctor, a little at a time. He also asks her more about her relationships in her family. Is her daughter supportive? What does she talk about with her daughter? Caroline admits she spends most of the time with her daughter complaining about her fatigue and pain. She even realizes that she massages her hands more when around her daughter than when she is by herself. "How do you think you might feel better while you're around your daughter and spend more time feeling better in general?" asks the psychiatrist. Caroline answers, "Maybe we could spend time doing fun things, like seeing a movie, or shopping."

Caroline takes these ideas to heart, and has a long talk with her daughter about what she's been feeling since her daughter moved away. They decide to plan phone calls and fun visits as the psychia-

trist suggested. After a few weeks, Caroline is back to her usual morning walks. She feels more energetic, and her knees aren't as stiff as they used to be. She focuses on spending time doing things she enjoys rather than being disappointed by her limitations. She no longer tells herself how exhausted she is—instead, she congratulates herself on her walking. She begins to ask her friends about different retirement communities and starts to feel more excited about a smaller, tidy new home she could arrange to her liking.

Patients who have serious, chronic medical conditions, such as diabetes or cancer, often come to realize that their attitude is an important part of their treatment. We can learn from how they cope with ongoing discomfort and uncertainty. Many of these patients say they make a conscious decision to control the illness as much as possible, and not let the illness control them or their quality of life. They practice responsible self-management behaviors by learning which circumstances are apt to trigger symptoms and then avoiding or modifying these triggers. They distract their minds from worries, and they participate in meaningful activities that give them satisfaction as often as possible. They foster the attitude that since the condition is chronic and there are limits to available treatment, the best approach is to turn their efforts toward coping with symptoms. Just as we have to practice *thinking* positively, we have to practice *living* positively. You can reduce the symptoms of benign chronic conditions with this approach.

The Stress Response

Stress is another common situational factor, and it is one of the most important amplifiers of symptoms. Stress arises from life events, work, interpersonal situations, or secret worries. Stress can both amplify preexisting symptoms of any disorder and also produce its own set of symptoms. Obviously, any situation in which you experience stress can make your symptoms worse, just as Caroline's arthritis worsened when she was stressed at the doctor's office. Understanding stress better allows us to think differently about many bothersome symptoms and, in turn, alleviate them.

Have you felt severely stressed out in the past month? Almost everyone has! Stress causes physical distress in millions of people year in and year out. Such diverse symptoms as headaches, insomnia, nausea, tremor, and sweaty palms can all be caused by stress. It's a natural reaction, but why would we have a natural reaction that could hinder our ability to overcome what is making us stressed in the first place? Understanding exactly what stress is and how it affects symptoms can go a long way to decrease its negative effect on the body.

Stress is the perception of a threat or a dangerous uncertainty combined with the thought that your resources won't be adequate to deal with the threat. It is any situation that makes you feel helpless or overwhelmed. To put it more simply, stress is being involved in a fender bender, your child being sick or doing poorly in school, your parents fighting, or hassling with your landlord. All of these situations lead to a cycle of brain and hormone reactions that can cause physical symptoms.

Our brains are constantly taking in information from the environment and from internal sensations. We then evaluate what is happening based on this information and past experience. When we perceive that a situation might exceed our ability to cope with or control it, an emergency signal goes off in the hypothalamus of the brain—the beginning of the stress response. The hypothalamus triggers the sympathetic nervous system to respond to an emergency, making us faster and stronger. The signal travels down to the adrenal glands, where adrenaline and other chemicals and hormones are injected directly into the bloodstream.

We feel several changes very quickly: the heart pumps faster, our breathing rate and muscle tension increase, blood pressure rises, and the mind speeds up its processing of information. The stomach and intestines are given signals to stop digesting food so all energy can be devoted to getting away from the threat. This so-called fight-or-flight response contributes to our survival in a real emergency. However, during periods of prolonged, continuing stress, the fight-or-flight response can remain activated without beneficial effects and can ultimately cause physical problems. Prolonged muscle tension and other manifestations of the nervous system in overdrive can lead to nausea, headaches, teeth grinding, and the multitude of other symptoms associated with stress.

Why would being chased by a hungry lion and the mere memory of getting yelled at by the boss cause the same cascade of hormones and chemicals in our bodies and brains? Because the brain does not distinguish between an event that is actually happening to us and one that we are remembering, anticipating, or even just imagining. Even if we are just imagining a difficult situation that never actually happens, the fight-or-flight reaction will be triggered. Your heart races when you think a stranger is following you down a dark street whether or not it turns out that someone is actually there.

If your mind is drawn to a symptom that worries you several times this evening, your body may respond to that worry by going into defensive mode. One patient got severe stomach pains the moment he stepped into his office every morning. He never had pains on the weekend unless he was watching a television show that reminded him of work.

The stress signals listed in the exercises at the end of this chapter are specific examples of typical body responses. This information can be used to develop alternative explanations for your symptom and point you in a direction that is more likely to reduce or relieve it.

The stress reaction itself causes symptoms that are disturbing and unpleasant all on their own. Those sensations of muscle tension and increased heart rate can then become the focus of attention and worry. In addition, stress also affects our perception of other symptoms and causes us to amplify them—it makes us quicker to conclude that an ambiguous sensation is not normal and might be a symptom or progression of a disease. Because most people know that stress is bad for health, once they're under stress, they're quicker to conclude that they've gotten sick or that their medical condition is worsening. Consider the example of a man who had been working a lot of overtime. He told his friends, "This job will give me a heart attack!" When he felt a burning in his chest, he quickly assumed the pain was in his heart—when the pain was much more likely to be from indigestion caused by his fourth cup of strong coffee that day.

Finally, stress can produce symptoms by aggravating a preexisting chronic disease. Thus, in a classic study, illnesses and symptoms among navy personnel after deployment were predicted by how much life stress they had undergone *before* the deployment. It is important to remember, however, that stress is not as powerful a precipitant of illness as most people think. Indeed, most people undergoing major life stress remain healthy. Therefore, other factors are important in determining whether stress makes various diseases worse. These include people's flexibility, resilience, openness to change, and the presence of social support systems.

There are two types of stress that are relevant to how we perceive our bodily symptoms. First, there are daily hassles and minor irritants, like traffic jams and barking dogs and telemarketers and noisy neighbors. For example, workers who feel that their jobs are too demanding, that they have less autonomy, more job insecurity, and less camaraderie with their coworkers, all report more lower back pain than workers who don't feel that way. Second, there are major life changes and events that are less frequent but that require large readjustments on our part, such as divorce, legal problems, and changing jobs. People report more symptoms and go to the doctor much more after losing their jobs, having to declare bankruptcy, or moving away to a new part of the country.

Sometimes a single major stressor can cause an ongoing problem. Jack Barnes never had heart palpitations until after his wife died suddenly in a car accident. The palpitations that he felt for the first time when the policemen told him the devastating news recurred for years and sent him to the emergency room half a dozen times.

The good news about stress is that it can be relieved without medicines, alcohol or other drugs, or quitting your job. The relaxation exercises taught in Chapter 3 cause a cascade of hormones and neurochemicals that work to reverse the changes brought on by stress. These natural relaxation hormones lower blood pressure, quiet pressured thinking, and bring on a sense of contentment and well-being. Once you have relaxed, you can begin to use your mind to help you relieve your symptoms rather than having thoughts that make your symptoms worse.

Learning about what contexts and situations cause you stress is a major step in learning to cope with ongoing symptoms. The following exercises will help you figure out where circumstances and stress are affecting you, and help you develop plans for change.

Exercises

1. How does context shape your perceptions?

Look at the following optical illusions:

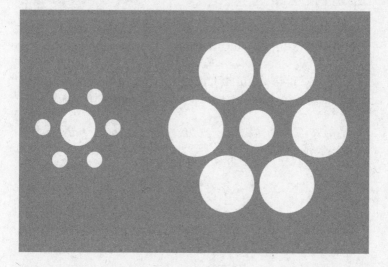

The two inner circles are actually the same size; it is the size of the circles surrounding them that influences how big you think they are. How large something seems depends on the context it is in.

How about the following drawing?

Do you see a white vase or the gray profiles of two people facing each other? We can change our perception of this picture if we change our vantage point. (You can try the same trick by looking at the maple leaf of the Canadian flag and see instead two angry men butting heads.)

2. Here is another exercise to illustrate how powerfully context can limit our perceptions:

      •   •   •

      •   •   •

      •   •   •

Can you connect all the dots using only four straight lines? (You can't cross the same dot with more than one line.)

Most people don't come up with the solution because they don't take a wider, broader view of the problem. They see it in too narrow a context. Here is the solution:

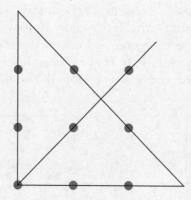

The answer involves extending the lines outside the limits of the figure—it involves, literally, "thinking outside the box." Things can look very different when you adopt a wider viewpoint.

3. Learn how your symptoms are affected by interpersonal relationships.

Write down how your symptom feels when you are alone, with a favorite person, or with a difficult person. Do you notice any patterns? How can you use what you've learned about your symptoms and interpersonal relationships to cope better with your symptoms?

4. Create your ideal situation.

Where do you feel best? Alone in your living room chair, or with your friends? Reading a book or watching an interesting television show? Write down an ideal situation, such as fishing with friends, enjoying an outdoor concert, or vacationing at the beach, then note how your symptoms would feel. Now write down an everyday situation, such as waking up in the morning. How do your symptoms feel? Write down a stressful situation, such as sitting in traffic. Are your symptoms worse? How can you achieve the good feelings of the ideal situation in an everyday situation? How can you let go of some of the stress in the stressful situation? Write down as many

Date/Time	Situation	Symptom	Current response: How did you handle the situation? Did it make your symptoms better or worse?	Expectation: What did you think would happen?	New response: Write ideas for responses that would take your mind off symptoms.
May 1, 4 p.m.	Boss tells me I'm working late.	Stomach upset	Told boss not feeling well. He didn't care. Indigestion and nausea worse. Angry, but can't risk job.	Thought boss would excuse me if not well. Thought he would remember I worked late twice last week.	Take break for light snack to settle stomach. Try to negotiate comp time next week. Focus on getting job done ASAP.
May 2, 2 p.m.	Doctor is short with me and tells me to see a therapist.	So tired	Angry that I didn't tell my doctor how I felt about what she said. Felt more exhausted and my arthritis hurts!	Hoped my doctor would listen patiently and tell me exactly what is wrong with me!	Tell my doctor how I felt, ask for her best explanation for my fatigue. Concentrate on feeling better, not being cured.

ideas as you can, and carry the best ones with you on a card to practice the next time you get stuck in a traffic jam.

5. Fill out a context worksheet at least once a day this week, modeling the two examples on the previous page. Keep track of how situations and circumstances affect your symptoms and personal feelings.

6. *Learn about stress.*

Take a moment to go through the stress signals list below. Identify any symptom that could be a manifestation of a stress response in you. What is going on in your life that might be stressful? What ideas do you have for a better way to deal with this situation? Try to follow Caroline's example to journal about how stress affects your symptoms at least once each day this week.

Physical Signals of Stress

Muscle tightness	Headache
Palpitations	Nervous tics
Dry mouth	Gastrointestinal problems
Being easily startled	Hyperventilation
Sweating	Chest tightness
Fatigue	Rash/hives
Insomnia	Weakness
Appetite change	Heavy legs

Behavioral Signals of Stress

Smoking	Overuse of alcohol or other drugs
Overeating	Arguing
Accident-prone	Teeth grinding

Emotional and Cognitive Signals of Stress

Anxiety/nervousness	Agitation
Irritability/anger	Depression
Restlessness	Forgetfulness
Nightmares	Frustration
Insecurity	Sharp mood swings
Ruminative thoughts	Apathy

Caroline's Workbook for Exercise Six

April 20: My pain worsened after my daughter moved farther away. It used to be that I could go and see her almost every weekend—now it takes planning and a long drive. Besides noticing my pain more, I've also been having other symptoms of a stress response. I'm clenching my teeth more, especially in the car on the way to the doctor's office. I'm more anxious overall, and I've been tired lately. Maybe I can spend more time with other friends, now that my daughter is gone.

April 22: Judith and I set up a card game with some of the other women at my church. It was a lot of fun, and helped me to unwind a little. My jaw isn't as tight, and my arthritis actually feels a little better. Also, I didn't notice it much at all while I was playing cards. This is a good sign!

April 25: Today I tried something new—my daughter and I set up a time each week where we have a long phone call. That way,

I know we can have some quality time together, and I won't worry about bothering her while she's in the middle of something else, since she is awfully busy. I noticed this week I worried about her less, and felt a little happier overall, knowing I would have the opportunity to tell her about my week and hear about her week too. I had no idea that her moving away had been so stressful for me—and that the stress was making my arthritis symptoms worse! Ever since I've been working on my stress, and trying to lessen the stress in my life, my arthritis and fatigue have definitely been better.

7. Imagine changing your circumstances and situations.

If you could change one stressful situation or interaction, what would it be? Think of ways to change your part in the situation, either by changing your perspective, your reactions, or the circumstances themselves.

8. Continue your relaxation practice!

Lie on your bed, face up, with your hands resting by your hips. Take a deep breath in through your nose, feeling your abdomen rise. When you have fully inhaled, keep taking in air until the column of breath reaches the back of your teeth. Then hiss, forcing all the air out through a small space between the top of your tongue and the roof of your mouth. Repeat five to ten times. If you like this exercise, try it every night before you go to sleep. You might be surprised how much deep breathing can lead to a good night's rest. You can count this breathing as part of the twenty minutes you should set aside almost every day for relaxation while you are doing the six-week program.

9. Bring relaxation into your everyday life.

Try to use mindfulness or relaxation at every opportunity. If driving to the store makes you tense and unhappy, take five minutes at your destination point to unwind. For example, go to the candles section of the grocery store and smell your favorite ones; close your eyes to really experience the pleasant sensations.

*   *   *

In this chapter, we've seen that the severity of a symptom is influenced by the situations we are in when we experience it. Situations, circumstances, and events provide clues to how we should interpret the symptom, how significant we think it is, and what it might mean (in particular, how serious it might be). Our circumstances also suggest to us what we should expect to feel next, and in this way they may contribute to a symptom getting worse. Interactions with other people, our relationships with our loved ones, and stressful events are all good examples of situations that can either amplify or alleviate symptoms. We've learned key skills in managing symptoms better: first, learn to identify the particular settings and events that make us feel worse, and alter them; second, cultivate the situations that make us feel better.

CHAPTER SIX

Week 4—Undo the Damage of Unproductive Behaviors

We've talked about the ways in which expectations, situations, and our thoughts about symptoms can make them better or amplify them. Another way to make symptoms feel better or worse is through our behavior. How we react to our symptoms, what we do with our time, and how we interact with others affects how we feel. Recognizing and then changing unproductive behaviors can be one of the most powerful ways to better cope with symptoms like cramps, dizziness, insomnia, and many others.

People who suffer from chronic symptoms often unintentionally behave in counterproductive ways that make their symptoms more pronounced and troublesome. These can include:

- avoiding usual or fun activities and coddling themselves unnecessarily;

- seeking more and more medical tests in order to feel more in control, and also seeking excessive reassurance from doctors; and

- researching medical conditions too much, whether by reading about them, asking others their opinions, watching TV, or using the Internet.

We engage in these kinds of behaviors for good reason—we believe they will keep us safe or make us feel better. While many of these health- and illness-related activities are beneficial when done in moderation, they can make things worse when we overdo them. Each of the behaviors listed above can be helpful up to a point. But it is also possible to engage in them so excessively that they end up amplifying our symptoms.

It is important to be an informed and educated patient—to know about your condition, monitor it, know when to consult your doctor, and understand your treatment. But it is possible to spend too much time and energy (and too much money) seeking medical tests and medical attention that really are unnecessary. Likewise, you can become overinvolved in your health by spending too much time reading about it, researching it on the Internet, and discussing it with others. When this happens, you can actually make your symptoms worse and impair your sense of well-being. Why? Well, as natural and prudent as it seems to learn as much as possible about your symptom or disease, all that time spent on the Internet or in the bookstore is *time spent feeling sick*. It is important to be well informed and proactive about your health without becoming so involved that you engage in maladaptive and unhelpful behaviors.

How do you know if you're overdoing it? When do these behaviors become excessive? Simple: the behavior is excessive if it adds to your distress. Your doctor tells you not to worry, that your clinical condition has not changed, and other trusted people say you don't look any worse. Perhaps you feel better after they reassure you, but soon suspicion creeps back in. You begin to think the doctor must have missed something, or your friend couldn't possibly know enough about the situation. Maybe you forgot to mention a symptom to the doctor or didn't give him or her a clear enough picture. Maybe the doctor didn't hear all that you said. Maybe the normal laboratory test results were erroneous, or there is a more sensitive test that wasn't done. You make more appointments, but feel a sense of disappointment and no more reassured each time. This kind of behavior takes time away from your regular activities, and there is nothing to be gained from repeating it. It is more *time spent feeling sick*.

We will explore each behavior in turn and explain how it can have the paradoxical effect of making the symptom worse. Ellen Farraday is a good example.

Ellen became concerned with her health when her best friend Sally was diagnosed with breast cancer. Fortunately, the lump was found early, and Sally had a good chance of being cured. Ellen had reason to be concerned, however, because her own mother died of breast cancer in her forties. Ellen always examined her breasts in the shower every month, without fail. Now that Sally had been stricken too, Ellen went onto the Internet to learn more about the inheritance of breast cancer, and about mammograms and any blood tests she might take to catch cancer in its earliest stages. With two young daughters, she had a good reason to make sure she was in the best of health. Sometimes she got so upset about Sally and worried about her own future that she stayed home from her daughters' soccer games.

Avoiding Usual Activities

Do you ever avoid activities, such as exercise or going out, that seem to make your symptoms worse? The question is a no-brainer—most people avoid doing things that seem to make their symptoms worse. Often, however, people avoid these activities not just because of the actual physical discomfort associated with the activity, but because they mistakenly believe that the physical discomfort indicates that the activity is harmful.

For example, many chronic fatigue syndrome sufferers restrict their activities because they believe that exertion worsens their disease; but studies have shown this is incorrect. In fact, a gradual, sustained program of progressive exercise is the best approach to this condition.[1] Inactivity only worsens the fatigue by allowing muscles to become weaker, decreasing exercise tolerance, and actually increasing feelings of fatigue and exhaustion.

Likewise with chronic pain: though a particular activity may intensify chronic pain, this does not mean that the activity is damaging to your body. Sudden, *acute* pain (such as a burn or a sprain) signals you that tissue has been injured and that you should cease whatever you are doing that is painful in order to prevent further damage. *Acute* pain alerts you that something is wrong and prompts you to take self-protective action. But *chronic* pain is a different story. Chronic pain, such as lower back pain, chronic headaches, or chronic pelvic pain, generally does not reflect ongoing tissue damage and therefore should not prevent exercise. Quite to the contrary, exercise is increasingly recommended for chronic pain patients. Even for people with chest pain from coronary heart disease, a graduated, supervised exercise program is the keystone of cardiac rehabilitation programs.

Inactivity makes your muscles weaker and your joints less flexible, which makes you stiffer and makes exercise even more painful. If a patient experiences symptoms while engaged in a particular activity, he may incorrectly assume that the activity caused the symptom, and decide to avoid that activity. However, since the symptom was not actually related to the activity, limiting participation only leads to other problems. The consequences of avoiding some activities can sometimes even make the problem worse. Deconditioning from inactivity adds to the perception of being weak and sick. In addition, a more sedentary lifestyle often leads to gaining weight, which puts more stress on muscles and joints.

David Moss decided to get more exercise by walking up the stairs to his office rather than taking the elevator. The first week he felt short of breath and his heart was drumming in his chest. He concluded that he might be stressing his heart too much and that he should protect himself by taking the elevator from then on. In fact, his heart was fine—except for being out of shape. That is what caused his breathlessness and rapid heartbeat in the first place, and avoiding exercise will only make his symptoms worse! Not only that, he will become more worried about having a weak heart.

One of the main hazards of avoidance is that you can never prove your assumption wrong and reassure yourself about the safety of participating. Laura Cathety had multiple sclerosis, and used to exercise on the treadmill at the YMCA. When she felt off balance, she told herself, "I'm going to fall and break my neck if I keep doing the treadmill. I can't exercise with my MS." She gave up exercising, then felt weaker and more tired, symptoms of both deconditioning and multiple sclerosis. At the advice of her doctor, she tried resuming exercise—beginning with the stationary bike, and then a treadmill with side rails. It turned out that the balance problem could be solved if she had side rails and used a moderate speed. She ended up proving to herself that she felt better when she was fit.

What have you given up for your symptoms? What activities have you stopped participating in? Ask your doctor if they are truly harmful to your health. If you are aware of a particular fear that limits a given activity, try facing that fear and figuring out the chance of the fear actually coming true. Use the exercises at the end of the chapter to conduct your own behavioral experiment; you can test if your observations about your symptoms are indeed related to the activity. If you are proved incorrect, you can safely resume this activity, and we provide a guide to help you do this. (Of course, as we've cautioned repeatedly throughout this book, we're only talking about symptoms that your doctor has thoroughly evaluated and treated, and for which he or she has told you that the activity is not dangerous.)

First, however, we have to examine another kind of common behavior that makes symptoms worse. In the previous chapter, we discussed how communication styles and family responses can provide a setting that amplifies your symptoms. Sometimes you might receive special consideration or support or can avoid some unpleasant activity because you're not feeling well. It's always nice to have others help you out or avoid situations that are unpleasant, but this can make it harder to resume these activities later on. So, while it makes sense to let others help you do something when you're feeling ill, it ultimately can make the symptom harder to control.

Charlotte Mendenhall was invited to attend her sister-in-law's wedding. She dreaded the wedding because she felt shy and inferior to her husband's family. On the morning of the wedding, she woke up with the splitting headache and nausea she often felt when facing family gatherings like these. After she told her husband how sick she felt, he agreed that she should stay home. She spent the day in bed and felt better by evening. But when her husband returned, they had an argument because he was irritated about attending the wedding alone. Her tension level increased and the headache returned. She made the connection that her fears led to the physical symptoms, and her behavior only made the problem worse in the long run. She decided it was time to break the pattern and address the real problem of boosting her self-confidence in social situations.

Examining Yourself Excessively and Seeking Too Much Reassurance from Doctors

Ellen begins checking her breasts every two weeks, then every week. When her friend Sally returns to the doctor with another lump, Ellen starts to check herself during every shower. She pokes and prods until her breasts are sore and bruised, and she wonders if the swelling and tenderness are signs of an inflammatory type of breast cancer she has read about. She checks under her arms and around her collarbone and neck for lymph nodes. When she finds a tiny one, she prods it until it is also sore. Now she is certain she has breast cancer and can't sleep because she's thinking about it. Sally is in the hospital for chemotherapy, and Ellen visits her. Ellen feels she can't burden her sick friend with her fears, but Sally senses something is wrong and asks Ellen why she looks so uncomfortable. Ellen bursts into tears. Sally convinces Ellen to go to the doctor for a complete checkup.

Paying close attention to an unpleasant sensation has been proven to intensify that sensation. Concentrate on the dryness of your eyes for a minute. Is there a tickle there, or a scratchy sensation? Would it help to rub them? Try it—you might find the sensation is even worse now. Focusing on an unpleasant sensation will intensify it, and we can sometimes make the irritation worse with the action we think will relieve it. Imagine you feel a lump in your throat—then repeatedly clear it. Do this enough, and you'll end up with a sore throat. Using your left hand more than usual because your right hand aches will cause

soreness in the left hand, since it's not used to perform-
ing so many actions. Repeatedly feeling a suspicious swelling in the neck bruises the tissue, makes the area tender,
and makes the swelling worse. Anxiety increases along
with the suspicion that there is a tumor growing in the
swollen area. Fear leads to heightened sensitivity and incorrect attributions, and the cycle of symptom amplification continues.

A common belief is that the only way to rule out a
condition is with a test. Shawn Bradley, a thirty-year-old
bus driver, was very concerned about prostate cancer. He
had read in a popular magazine that he should ask his
doctor about a special test for it. Even though he had no
signs of the disease, and he was so young it would be very
rare for him to have prostate cancer, his doctor gave in to
his request and ordered the test. The physician thought
there was no chance of a positive result, but hoped that a
negative test result would reassure Shawn that he didn't
have cancer. But paradoxically, Shawn concluded that because the doctor had agreed to go through with the test,
the doctor must suspect that he really did have cancer.
When the result was negative, Shawn was not reassured.
His anxiety led him to a common belief: that while positive results are reliable, negative results are not.

Here's another example of this process at work: Carl
returned from vacation feeling refreshed and healthy. A
few days later, he read in the newspaper that a strain of
encephalitis had been found in the area where he had
vacationed. He became worried. He thought he felt a
bit feverish and noticed he had a headache. He called his
doctor, requesting a blood test. The doctor reviewed his
chances of exposure, explained the incubation time and
usual warning signs, and said that if Carl still felt ill he
would do the test even though he thought the chances of
Carl developing encephalitis were negligible. Carl waited

the length of time necessary for exposure to be detectable, and then had the blood test. The test was negative, but Carl only worried more, fearing the lab was unfamiliar with the test, or that he had an unusual strain of encephalitis that would not register. When Carl's headaches persisted, he returned to the doctor and was diagnosed with tension-type headaches brought on by the worrying about the encephalitis. Studies of people with chest pain and with abdominal complaints have shown that, among those who are anxious about their health to begin with, a negative diagnostic test is not reassuring and they continue to worry in spite of a normal test result.[2] So if you're anxious about a symptom to start with, a normal laboratory test result may not reassure you.

Often patients underestimate the danger of complications of invasive tests, and put themselves at risk from the test itself. There is much debate in medical circles about the value of many standard medical tests used for screening and diagnosis. There are risks to investigating your symptoms, just as there are risks to ignoring them. The risks can include adverse reactions to medications or contrast material given for tests, injuries during the procedure, prolonged discomfort from the test, and cumulative exposure to radiation from X-rays. You will benefit from a frank discussion with your primary care physician about the need for, limitations, and risks of diagnostic procedures.

In the face of chronic, benign conditions, the time finally comes to halt testing and focus more on getting on with one's life. At some point, pursuing fruitless diagnostic procedures and undergoing radical, expensive, and hazardous treatments just serve to distract you from learning to cope with your illness, from minimizing your symptoms and learning to compensate for them. As long as you expect that you will ultimately find a cure, you don't truly accept that you're going to have to make the most of your condition, and you don't develop the coping skills and strategies that would allow you to overcome it. In addition, there are other risks involved in overaggressive treatment of conditions that are uncomfortable but aren't terribly serious. These risks include experiencing medication side effects, developing resistance to antibiotics or rebound pain from pain medications, becoming weaker from unnecessary activity restrictions, and having secondary problems like missing work or family obligations. By asking the question "How might I try to improve my situation regardless of my medical condition?" the door is opened for improving your quality of life.

Ellen and her primary care physician discuss Ellen's risk factors for breast cancer. She does have an increased risk due to her mother's illness, but no other relatives have the disease. She is thirty-two, and breast cancer at such a young age is very rare. Ellen wants a mammogram, but her doctor warns her that mammograms in young women are difficult to read and have false-positive results more often than in older women. Indeed, if the chances of Ellen actually having a cancer are very small, a positive test is more likely to be a false positive than a true positive. False-positive mammograms can lead to unneeded biopsies, which cause pain, scarring, and can be complicated by infection. Ellen's doctor does not feel any suspicious lumps and wants Ellen to wait a few years before her first mammogram.

We seek reassurance in many direct and indirect ways. Direct ways include asking family members or friends, "How do you think I look?" Perhaps you call your physician to report that the flu symptoms have improved and wait for her to say, "You'll be fine now." There are indirect ways to seek reassurance: sneaking references to health into a store checkout lane conversation, scanning magazine articles that explain which symptoms indicate serious disease. You might ask an aunt, "Can lightheadedness be caused by multiple sclerosis? Does MS run in our family? Did you ever know anyone with MS?" When she replies she had a coworker who did develop MS, it confirms your suspicion that the disease is common, and your fear that it is the cause of your lightheadedness.

Think back to a recent doctor's appointment. Did you feel reassured after the visit? How long did the reassurance last? What usually happens when you go to the doctor? Some of you may notice that even when you get the response you thought you wanted, the reassured feeling doesn't last for long. The worries creep back in, and you may question or disregard what was said. Anxious people replay the visit over and over, worrying they did not convey their situation accurately, so the doctor didn't get the right picture. Or perhaps the doctor wasn't paying sufficient attention to the patient's history, or simply forgot to order a test that was indicated. Anxiety creeps up right after feeling better.

Have there been times when you sought reassurance to feel less worried and it backfired? When you have symptoms, whom do you consult? Try to use the techniques in this book to convince yourself of an alternative, benign interpretation of your observations before you seek more information *for symptoms that have already been examined by your doctor.*

Ellen sets up an appointment with another doctor, who agrees to let Ellen have a mammogram. The waiting list for the test is a month long, and then one long week passes before the radiologist is able to read it. In the meantime, Sally has completed her chemotherapy and seems cancer-free for the time being. Sally is happy to be out of the hospital and spending time with her friends and family. Ellen is fretful and depressed, waiting for

the mammogram results to come back. She is almost certain it
will be positive for cancer. She now checks her breasts twice a day,
and the soreness is always present.

Researching Medical Conditions

We all need to be informed consumers and active
participants in our own health care. However, there is a
limit to the type and amount of information that is beneficial. Remember the example of the "medical student
syndrome"? Often, reading medical books or browsing
the Internet for research studies or support groups ex-
poses people to misinformation that can heighten disease fears and lead to misinterpreting perfectly harmless
sensations in new and frightening ways.

Rhonda Green spent an inordinate amount of time
looking up her prescription medications in the *Physician's Desk Reference,* and worrying about potential side
effects. Before long, the power of suggestion took hold,
and she began to feel some of the side effects listed.
Studies with placebo pills have shown this power of suggestion. One-quarter of people taking a placebo pill
develop side effects. Just believing that they are taking a
powerful drug with serious side effects leads people to
mistakenly think that preexisting symptoms they never
much noticed before are due to the new drug. The amaz-
ing fact, however, is that they're only taking a sugar
pill.

It is now standard practice for pharmacists to en-
close a comprehensive printout of drug information
with each prescription. But telling people about possible
side effects tends to lead them into experiencing the
side effects. A research study using aspirin for heart
problems that was conducted at two different hospitals

ran into this unexpected effect.[3] One hospital required that the patients be given full printouts about potential side effects that included a specific warning about possible gastric distress. Their patients reported gastric distress as a side effect *six times* more often than the patients at the hospital that did not give out such detailed information.

Getting into the habit of researching every symptom can lead to overlooking commonsense explanations in your quest of the more exotic. As Ann Landers once wrote, "Be careful what you read about health. You could die of a misprint." The media contribute to many fears by selecting a "disease of the month" and reporting on it in a sensationalistic way. Sometimes the statistics quoted are inaccurate, or studies cited are taken out of context or apply only to a small population. It is wise to regard health information you get on TV, over the radio, and through magazines with a bit of suspicion and to bring the information you are curious about to your doctor. If something about your condition or its treatment particularly worries you, ask your doctor directly about your misgivings or uncertainties. Going from one doctor to another hoping that you'll find one who just happens to guess what's troubling you and address your unspoken fears can lead to even more worry, waiting, and pain.

Ellen's mammogram results are negative, but she has read in a magazine about people whose cancers were accidentally missed. One of the members of a breast cancer Web site she frequents had a sister who died after a radiologist's oversight. Ellen returns to the doctor with the names of top radiologists she would like to have read her mammogram. She is beginning to feel as if she has a death sentence of cancer looming. Sally asks Ellen to go back to her original primary care physician, who has known

Ellen for years, in the hopes that she can alleviate Ellen's fears. Sally asks her own cancer specialist to give Ellen's doctor a call.

Changing Health Behaviors

When we talk about changing health behaviors and developing coping strategies, we mean two major types of change:

- starting or resuming activities that pose no threat to health; and
- eliminating behaviors that perpetuate symptoms.

Our focus is to help you feel better, not to search for an illsory cure.

Ellen's doctor looks at the mammogram in the office. She tells Ellen again that the risks of her having cancer are negligible, and lets her know that she has spoken to Sally's cancer specialist, who agrees. Ellen's doctor says frankly that Ellen's worrying is ruining her life. She asks Ellen if getting the mammogram made her feel better, and Ellen admits it did not. The doctor asks if the process of checking her breasts so often makes her feel better or worse. Ellen says she feels worse. The doctor writes out a list of pleasant, distracting activities, and tells Ellen she has to do at least one a day to get her mind off her health for a little while. She schedules a follow-up appointment in one month to check in on how Ellen is doing.

Starting or Resuming Healthy Activities

Maintaining an active life while pacing yourself can be a challenge. Think about an activity that you now avoid but used to enjoy before your symptoms became problematic. It might be physical exercise, social events, or taking care of your home. Resuming that activity can help boost your confidence by giving you back some control over the symptom. Keep your expectations realistic—if you have stopped taking walks, the lack of exercise may have left you in a deconditioned state, so don't expect to go back to full capacity right away. Be patient with yourself as you rebuild endurance. Take note of how your symptom feels before and after the activity. Take on a new challenge in small steps. For example, if before you stopped exercising you used to walk four blocks to the store, set a goal of two blocks and start by going out for a half-block stroll. Plan a reward in advance to recognize your accomplishment and reinforce the healthy new behavior. You deserve it!

If you have withdrawn from socializing because you don't feel well, pick a person you would like to see again. Call up a friend and make a date to have lunch together. Keep the conversation away from medical issues and focus on enjoying the company, surroundings, and food. When that feels comfortable, select a community or entertainment event that catches your interest and invite that friend to accompany you. After the event, check in on your symptoms. Remember that you are working on changing the belief that this activity makes your symptoms worse by proving to yourself that there is no causal connection. In fact, you will more likely feel better after enjoying yourself.

Jen Ross described withdrawing from her weekly bridge club meetings because she felt embarrassed by the unattractive red patches on her skin from psoriasis. Her embarrassment kept her from meeting anyone in public, and she only told her closest friend, Catie, who had suffered from eczema in the past. Because Jen's condition made such an impact on her life, she needed to express her feelings and experiences, but she realized that much of her time spent with Catie was spent talking about Jen's health. Jen decided to try branching out. She picked up Catie for an evening out and suggested new ground rules. She would not mention her illness the whole evening, and Catie would agree not to ask her about it. Jen had a new and enjoyable experience without the focus on illness. She discovered that she and Catie shared an interest in art, and they planned an excursion to the art museum. Jen was momentarily aware of her skin, but the thought passed when she turned her focus away from herself and onto the animated conversation.

Roger Dalton had suffered from diabetes for years, and it caused a painful condition in his feet. They burned and tingled most of the day, and his doctor told him there was little that could be done after a few medications known to help had failed to relieve the sensation. Depressed, Roger stopped golfing, something he used to love. He would sit in the house all weekend with his feet up, and the burning kept getting worse. Fed up with Roger's moping around, his best friend Dave set up a tee time. They drove the course instead of walking it, and Roger realized by the end of the day that he hardly spent any time thinking about his feet, and they felt better than when he spent the whole day in the house.

When a person has been in the "sick person" role in the family, other members often take over that person's responsibilities. Is there a responsibility or family function that you have relinquished because of your condition but feel motivated to take back? Let your family know your plan, then pace yourself as you regain control of the activity that is important to you. If you have turned over the cooking to your husband, you might plan to prepare dinner one night a week to start. Begin with simpler meals and ask a family member to do the cleanup that night. As you notice your symptoms do not become worse and your energy increases, you will convince yourself that cooking is not harmful to your health. Quite to the contrary, a positive consequence will be that you can take back more of the responsibilities that give you satisfaction and control.

Pleasurable activities are all the little things that give life meaning and enjoyment. We need to deliberately seek out and engage in these pleasurable activities every day as a way of taking time for ourselves, as a buffer against stress, and as an energy boost. Pleasurable activities are both planned and spontaneous. Examples include walking in a park, tending plants, having an uninterrupted cup of tea, feeding birds, baking cookies, looking through an old photo album, watching children at the playground, and so on. What pleasurable activities have you tried lately?

Since you're bothered by uncomfortable and unpleasant physical sensations—your symptoms—it's particularly important to discover and cultivate other sensations and sensory experiences that are enjoyable and pleasurable. There are pleasurable physical sensations such as massage, dancing, a hot bath, or exercising; there are auditory experiences like listening to music or the sound of rain or waves on a beach; there are the joys of great-tasting food and pleasing aromas like baking bread, flowers, and perfume; and there are visual experiences like art, interior design, and sunsets.

Eliminating Behaviors That Perpetuate Symptoms

An easy way to pick apart and examine the behaviors that make us feel better or worse is to start with the

ABCs. Antecedents, "A," are the circumstances that set the stage for behaviors. An example might be that you feel achy and irritable. Behaviors, "B," are what you do in response to the antecedent. When you feel achy, you might curl up on the couch with some chocolate bonbons and complain to a family member about how terrible you feel. Consequences, "C," are what results from the behaviors. Your spouse may offer to do the laundry and pick up the house, without any help from you. Unfortunately, this sequence, very likely to happen in a supportive family, reinforces negative coping behaviors. Instead of engaging in an activity that might be distracting or enjoyable, you sit on the couch feeling sick and eat far too many bonbons.

Compare that sequence to the following: A=you notice that your back is aching. B=you ask your spouse to join you in preparing dinner while you talk about pleasant subjects. C=you feel more satisfaction with yourself, so your mood improves and your back pain is less noticeable.

Other strategies to reduce or eliminate symptoms could include setting a time-out on reading medical articles that make you more nervous. You could try not reading about health-related topics for one week. If you check in on your pain level frequently, you might start reducing this by only allowing yourself to check in at the top of the hour. If you worry a lot about your illness, you might set a time for worrying, perhaps four in the afternoon for thirty minutes. During the day when your mind strays to worries, jot down the subject, and wait until four o'clock to worry. Use a problem-solving approach and keep this appointment even if the urge to worry has passed. After thirty minutes, get up and get busy with something else. This not only begins to curtail the behavior, but it also gives you some measure of control over it.

If you habitually examine yourself to check on your symptoms, you can set aside a specific time instead of doing it throughout the day. Then you can begin limiting the length of time you allow for self-examination. Doing this begins to give you some control over it. Very gradually over the weeks, keep decreasing the time you allow for examining yourself, and then space out these allotted times, making them less and less frequent. As a result you will feel less at the mercy of your illness and find that it bothers you less.

If you want to eliminate a behavior that elicits a response from others that makes your symptoms worse, focus directly on your behavior or communication. It is more realistic to change ourselves than to change someone else. Family responses will probably start to change as you change. And remember, changing a behavior may seem overwhelming at first; it is important to break up your larger goals into smaller ones and achieve one manageable bit at a time. Change must be accomplished very gradually, but you can make enormous strides over the long run if you do it in a series of small incremental steps forward, each of which is mastered in turn before going on to the next one.

Ellen is reassured by her primary care physician's assessment and advice. She spends more time with her family and friends and finds she does feel much better when she avoids the topic of health and cancer. Sally is pleased to see Ellen feeling better. When Ellen sees the doctor again, they talk once more about Ellen's frequent self-examination, which is painful and not helpful. Ellen agrees to try to cut down to twice a month. She also limits her reading and researching of breast cancer to a few hours on the weekend, and she makes sure that she looks up other things, such as current events or the weather, with most of the time she spends on the Internet. Occasionally she finds herself slipping back to checking herself more often than she should, or going to a breast cancer Web site on a weekday, but she does her best to refrain. She lives with the fear of cancer, and no longer allows it to take over her life.

Setting New Goals

Goals work best when they are phrased in a positive way, describe a specific behavior, and are measurable. Steps include:

- Select a long-term goal for six months from now.

- Break the long-term goal into short-term goals— steps you can take over the next few weeks and months.

- List the long-term goals and the short-term steps in a workbook.

- Remember that you can best make a major change in your behavior if you break your ultimate goal down into many small incremental steps. Master each small step completely before advancing to the next one. Aim for slow but steady progress toward your goal.

- Be patient and determined about reaching your goal. Practice one short-term step every day. Plan frequent rewards to reinforce your progress, and celebrate the healthy progress you are making.

- Everyone slips once in a while. Make sure your goal is realistic, figure out how to avoid the slip in the future, and then go right back to your plan.

Exercises

1. Identify problematic behaviors.

What is the first thing you do when you feel the symptom that bothers you most? Is this activity likely to help you feel better overall, or does it merely address the symptom and keep you from engaging in the activities you enjoy? Write down the behavior and all the negative and positive results from it.

Ellen's Workbook for Exercise 1

I feel sore in my left breast—the first thing I do is massage it to try to make the pain go away—but that often makes it feel even more tender. Other times I go to the Internet and look up information on breast cancer—that almost never makes me feel better.

2. How does your behavior impact others and how they treat you?

Imagine you have taped a typical evening at home when you are not feeling well, and you are watching the videotape without sound. How would someone else watching the tape know you felt sick? Describe your behavior and the message it sends to those around you. When we are in pain we might grimace, take a pill, limp, or rub the affected limb—all of these behaviors send nonverbal messages to those around us. How do they respond? Are there messages on both sides that would be healthier and more to your advantage?

3. Continue to practice relaxation or mediation for twenty minutes five times a week.

Here is another exercise to try: Change your computer monitor desktop to a beautiful landscape. Imagine you are in that place using every sense. What would it smell like? How would the air feel on your skin, or the ground feel beneath your feet? What sounds would you hear? What is the temperature?

4. Set goals to change problematic behaviors.

Make a list of specific behaviors that exacerbate your symptoms. You may include the behavior you used for Exercise 1. Put a star (*) next to the ones you would be interested in *changing*. How can changing this behavior be formulated into a goal?

Ellen's Workbook for Exercise 4

Behaviors that make my symptoms worse: * avoiding my friends and family because I'm so worried about dying. The other night, when my husband and I went out for dinner, we talked about pleasant things, and I felt better. I'll formulate a set of goals around that experience.

Long-term goal: I will not think so much about dying and breast cancer.

Short-term goal: I will spend twenty minutes of quality time with my husband each day for the next two weeks.

5. Put visits to the doctor in context.

Make a log to keep track of how often and why you are tempted to call your doctor. This can help you understand what circumstances and situations bother you most and make you want to reach out for more help or support or advice. In a log this week, keep track of the number of times you were tempted to call or e-mail your doctor and whether you feel worse or better while: (1) leaving a message, (2) waiting for the return call, (3) speaking with or getting a message from your doctor. Did communicating with the doctor help your symptoms? What was it about the discussion that was helpful—getting lab test results, being reassured, knowing that the doctor had spent some time thinking about you? Was the conversation not helpful? Why not? Was your doctor impatient, or did he or she not get back to you for several days while you worried?

There is nothing wrong with calling your doctor about medical symptoms. However, if calling the doctor is a primary mechanism you use to soothe your symptoms, it may be important to explore other ways you can feel better. When these other ways are less dependent on the schedule, mood, and abilities of another person, control over how you feel reverts back to you.

6. *Practice recognizing troublesome behaviors and learn aspects of what initiates them and how you can change them with the ABCs of the Behavior Worksheet on the next page. Make a copy in your workbook and fill one row at least once a day this week.*

7. *Do at least one pleasant activity every day! Here is a long list you can choose from. Be sure to add your own favorite things to do at the end.*

> *Play with cards, games, puzzles*
> *Help out in the community*
> *Soak in the bathtub with bubbles*
> *Add to your favorite collection*

Date	Symptom	Antecedents: How were you feeling? What was on your mind? What was going on?	Behaviors: How did you handle the situation?	Consequences: What happened? Did you feel better or worse?	Alternatives: How could you handle it differently next time?
Jan. 7	Breast pain	Feeling tired, ill. Kids fighting. Sally had just gone back to the hospital.	Checked Internet breast cancer chat room.	Learned about a new kind of radiation-resistant cancer. Felt much worse.	Go for a jog, check travel sites to plan a vacation, call my sister.
Jan. 9	Armpit aches	News was on—major car accident on the freeway, crime rate is rising. So much depressing news about the world today!	Felt the armpit repeatedly, looking for swollen lymph nodes, maybe a sign of cancer.	Armpit began to ache more, worried more about cancer.	Turn the TV off, help the kids with their homework, start dinner.
Jan. 11	Feeling tired	Didn't sleep well last night. Daughter Amanda kept waking me up with questions about her outfit for her dance recital. Tough day at the office.	I was stressed out and called Sally in the hospital—she mentioned how tired she was all the time.	Thought that my fatigue might be another sign that I have cancer.	Be proactive about getting good sleep, buy a new soft pillow, put a "Do Not Disturb" sign on the door—the kids are old enough to not need me at night except for emergencies.

Plan a weekend vacation
Go on a date
Fly a kite
Have sex
Sing out loud
Practice spirituality
Go to a movie in the middle of the week
Walk, jog, hike, skate, swim
Listen to music
Lie in the sun
Develop a plan to get ahead in your career
Put together a scrapbook of your last vacation photos
Pursue your favorite hobby—painting, beading,
*   needlepoint, carpentry*
Spend time with friends
Go camping, to the beach, or fishing
Play a musical instrument
Join a club
Buy clothes
Meet new people
Fix a gourmet meal
Repair something broken in your home
Remember kind words someone said about you
Garden, arrange flowers
Go to a play or concert
Play with children
Daydream

* * *

In this chapter, we learned how our actions can adversely affect our symptoms. Knowing about how behaviors cause us distress gives us the ability to modify them and feel better. You made note of many different behaviors, figured out which ones were causing you difficulty, and set goals to change them. Some of these goals can be chal-

lenging to meet, but you've already come a long way in
learning the best ways to cope with your symptoms. Like
Ellen, you can learn how to approach life differently and
spend much less time being worried or feeling ill. Keep
up the good work!

CHAPTER SEVEN

Week 5—Brighten the Mood, Help the Symptom

Moods and Symptoms

It is impossible to separate emotional and physical well-being. Have you ever noticed that your physical symptoms worsen when you are emotionally upset? A stomachache will get much worse if you top it off with an argument with your landlord, and the prospect of a stressful day ahead can make you feel as if you barely have the energy to open your eyes, much less get out of bed and get on with your day. You may tend to think that a bodily symptom has *either* a physical source *or* that it's "all in your head." But no bodily symptom is all in your head, and all symptoms have *both* a bodily component and a psychological component.

Emotional and physical discomfort go hand in hand, each serving to make the other worse. After you've been sick for a while, you can't help but get frustrated, demoralized, and irritable. Conversely, the feelings of anxiety, anger, guilt, depression, and low self-esteem often are accompanied by headaches, fatigue, loss of appetite, insomnia, and difficulty concentrating. Most of the time it is not clear which came first, the unhappiness or the physical symptoms. The truth is it doesn't matter! Symptoms and bad moods are an ongoing cycle in which each fuels the other in a continuous feedback loop.

Anxiety is one mood state that can worsen medical symptoms. The very word anxiety brings to mind tense shoulders, a sick feeling in the stomach, breaking into a sweat, heart pounding, and a dry mouth. Research has shown that anxious people are more sensitive to pain and have more visits to the doctor than those who are relaxed. Like anxiety, depression also magnifies physical discomfort. At one time or another, most people with chronic illnesses feel dejected and demoralized about their situation. Another common response to chronic symptoms is anger, and anger, too, can make symptoms worse.

In previous chapters, we discussed the stress response and how it causes bodily symptoms. We have charted examples when being under stress made physical symptoms worse. Certain emotions and moods, such as anxiety, depression, and anger, can also affect physical symptoms. Learning how to monitor moods and deal with them can decrease the distress and disability of chronic symptoms.

Anxiety

Anxiety is what we experience when we believe we are in danger or threatened. But the danger or threat doesn't have to be real. If you *think* you're about to be mugged in a dark alley, you will feel anxious whether or not the mugger is really there. Anxiety is a state of increased scrutiny, worry, and self-consciousness. It puts us on guard and makes us hypervigilant, constantly scanning our surroundings for some anticipated threat or danger. Anxious people are also more self-conscious and scrutinize themselves and their bodies more. All of these amplify symptoms and health concerns. Anxiety has its own set of bodily symptoms, too, which only add further to our misery.

Have you ever experienced the physical sensations of anxiety? Sometimes it may cause feelings of intense panic or impending doom, but many times it is experienced as a sensation of muscle tension, of being jittery, revved up, and unable to relax. Anxiety has a futuristic dimension—the apprehension that something bad is about to happen. Because we anticipate some kind of physical or emotional harm, our usual bodily discomforts feel worse. And anxiety can make even neutral sensations more annoying. Research on anxious people shows that they consider having their fingers lightly rubbed with sandpaper to be painful, while nonanxious people don't.[1]

When anxious, the mind is easily alarmed and on the lookout for internal and external threats—it's like a microphone listening to the body for faint but potentially dangerous signals that could indicate that something has gone wrong. Because anxiety makes us anticipate danger and harm, symptoms that we used to think were insignificant and trivial now become ominous and alarming portents of some ill-defined, impending disaster. Anxiety clouds our thinking, and we can distort health-related information and misperceive bodily sensations as more threatening than they really are. Our patient John Gibbons illustrated this point.

John's father died at age forty-three of a heart attack. Because of his family history, when John reached his forty-third birthday, he became a little more anxious about his health and thought he noticed some days that his heart was skipping a beat. He became quite concerned and began checking his pulse. The more he did this the more palpitations he noticed, and it also seemed that his heart was racing an awful lot. When he began surfing the Internet for information, he came across a warning about the increased danger of lethal, irregular heart rhythms if your resting heart rate was "above normal." This heightened his concern, and he finally went to see his doctor.

In the end, heart monitoring showed that he had only the occasional extra beats that every healthy person has, but his anxiety had increased his heart rate and made his palpitations seem more prominent and more frequent. Interestingly, John happened to revisit the same heart disease website afterward, and he discovered that his anxiety had caused him to misread the article in the first place: now he saw that the article actually said that the danger of arrhythmias was increased if your heart rate was "*way* above normal." He realized that in his earlier anxious state he had overlooked the word "way."

Anxiety also has direct effects on the body's nervous, endocrine, and cardiovascular systems. These changes themselves can easily be misinterpreted as worsening symptoms of a disease you already have or as symptoms of new disease. The physical effects of anxiety include a pounding or racing heart, muscle tension, sweating, flushing, and stomach churning. We're all familiar with the cold clammy hands, dry mouth, restlessness, and lump in the throat we feel before having to give a public talk or go into a meeting with our boss.

Anxiety also makes us tense up our muscles, and this increased muscle tone produces headaches, muscle soreness, and neck and shoulder pain. Try this experiment to prove the point: Hold out your hand, palm up, fingers outstretched. Then place a sheet of paper on your hand. The paper will quiver because it magnifies the normal, fine tremor that we all have in our hands. Now tense up the muscles in your arm and hand. The paper will show you how much worse the tremor becomes with tension.

When we're very anxious, we tend to breathe more rapidly. This changes the acid-base balance in the blood, which in turn causes numbness and tingling sensations, dizziness, and feeling faint. Anxious people are more tuned in to their body sensations and more easily alarmed, so that when these new physical symptoms of anxiety are added, they suspect that a new and ominous disease may be developing, or that a preexisting illness is worsening. The anxious person now has more physical symptoms to misinterpret as evidence of disease, which gives him more to worry about, which causes more physical symptoms...and the cycle goes round and round.

Some degree of anxiety is a normal and expected response to illness because being sick raises the specter of growing discomfort and disability, threatens our established relationships with family and friends, may affect our professional responsibilities and how others regard us, and may even jeopardize our ability to carry out the simple but important tasks of everyday life. But sometimes the anxious response can be excessive and we become overly concerned about our health status. Our illness concerns begin to distract us from our responsibilities to others and impair our ability to enjoy the pleasures of our day. At some point, if we become too preoccupied with our own health problems, we may begin to alienate and tax those who are close to us with our constant demands for assistance, sympathy, or reassurance.

Depression

Tony just isn't himself anymore. He used to be an easygoing guy who loved every moment of his job as a firefighter. However, a few months ago, one of his buddies was seriously burned on the job. Tony was present when it happened, but he was unable to keep his friend from being hurt. Ever since the accident, Tony has been more agitated and his mood has been terrible. Sometimes he doesn't want to get out of bed in the morning. He's felt more tired, his muscles ache, and his appetite suffers. He starts to worry that he's not strong enough to do his job and that he'll get injured—or, worse, that his weakness will cause someone else to be hurt. Worst of all, he no longer gets any enjoyment out of his life with his wife and son. Everyday things he used to think were fun don't matter to him anymore.

Tony begins to call in sick because he feels so lousy. He goes to his doctor wondering if he has some degenerative muscle condition like Lou Gehrig's disease. He used to run five miles a day, but now he doesn't have the energy, and he's afraid he will hurt himself. He becomes sad at the drop of a hat (for example, while watching some TV commercials) and increasingly worries that he'll end up in the hospital. He is plagued by financial worries and imagines that his son's college fund will have to be used for medical bills. When Tony's buddy from Ladder 32 goes back to work after recovering from his burns, Tony misses the welcome-back party.

Clinical depression is the experience of having a sad mood for most days for at least two weeks along with a loss of interest in the world around you. You become despondent and discouraged, lose your self-esteem, and find it harder and harder to have fun, enjoy yourself, and experience pleasure. You stop pursuing your hobbies, lose interest in playing cards or watching football on TV, and stop making social plans. You withdraw into yourself, become disinterested in those around you, and are preoccupied with your own distress. At any given time, about 10 percent of the population is clinically depressed. Twenty percent of women and a smaller number of men will experience depression during their lifetime.

The increased self-consciousness of depression is a

surefire recipe for amplifying symptoms. It magnifies pre-existing symptoms and causes us to focus on minor discomforts we'd previously ignored or dismissed, and makes them seem worse. This in turn makes our mood worse, and leads to a cycle of deepening depression and intensifying physical symptoms.

When we get depressed, we develop a negative view of ourselves and our future. We lose hope. A pessimistic outlook fosters the recall of unhappy memories and unpleasant past experiences, and a more negative appraisal of our health; we expect things to go badly. Not only do depressed people recall more negative than positive experiences, but they also remember these past experiences as worse than they actually seemed at the time. Depression causes people to feel weak and impaired, or as if they are being punished. They feel they don't deserve to be well and expect to be miserable. They dwell on painful memories and past illnesses and injuries, worry about becoming sicker, and think about death. The depressive outlook on life makes physical illness seem more pervasive and more overwhelming.

While lying alone in her dark room at night, Georgia Redding thinks back to a time when she was a child, recuperating from having her tonsils removed. She remembers feeling miserable and in pain. Now when she focuses on the burning in her throat from acid reflux disease, she fears that medical treatment will fail and she will get cancer in her esophagus like it says on the television commercials. Both the burning and the sense of helplessness intensify as she broods. When Georgia is not depressed, she remembers the same recuperation period from her childhood in a more favorable light; she even remembers it as a time when she was especially close to her mother, received presents from friends, and got special treats like ice cream. But her current depressed state colors her memories, worsening her perception of her current symptoms and intensifying her discomfort.

In addition to all of this, clinical depression has its own set of bodily symptoms. The common physical signs of depression include insomnia, constipation, loss of appetite, difficulty concentrating, and fatigue. These are distressing in themselves, but they are also often mistaken as evidence that one's physical illness is spreading or progressing.

Being in pain for a long time is enough in itself to cause depression. Ninety percent of chronic pain patients have symptoms of depression, and as many as half of them have a clinically significant depressive disorder. Conversely, most depressed patients report that physical symptoms (such as headaches, back and chest pain, and muscle aches) are among the things that bother them most. It is usually not clear what causes what—that is, whether their physical symptoms or their unhappy mood came first. Feeling sick makes you depressed and upset, and depression makes you feel sicker.

Anger

Anger is a common and powerful emotion that is a natural response to becoming sick. If harnessed correctly, anger can be very activating in our lives, helping us to be assertive, achieve our goals, and move forward. On the other hand, if anger is expressed in maladaptive ways, it can be frightening and destructive. Think back to times when you've been furious. Did you come into conflict with people around you? Did the anger help your situation, or make it worse by causing others to avoid you? What happened when you held your anger in? If it is not expressed at all, it can build up and lead to feelings of being sad, anxious, or overwhelmed.

Anger can be especially insidious in the case of chronic illness or symptoms. You want to curse your bad luck, get back at something. Unfortunately, the easiest and most accessible targets for your anger are the ones dearest to you—family, friends, and yourself. Anger can also lead to unhealthy behavior such as bouts of drinking, binging on unhealthy foods, resuming smoking, or not taking prescribed medications.

Tony's wife is very worried about how he has been doing, and asks him lots of questions about his sitting in his room all day, and the days of work he's missed. He hears her questions as criticism rather than concern, and it really gets on his nerves. After a while, every time his wife talks about anything remotely related to him, he tenses up and responds sharply, "Get off my back!" He's started slamming doors to end arguments. A couple of times he even thought about punching the wall.

Managing Moods

There are a number of ways to manage anxiety, depression, and anger. Some strategies to reduce anxiety include physical exercise, relaxation exercises, taking direct action to solve the things you are worried about, postponing your worries until a specific prearranged time later in the day, distracting yourself, keeping thoughts in the present moment with meditation, or engaging in a pleasurable activity.

Anxiety about health issues is often made worse by "catastrophizing." This means misinterpreting an uncomfortable bodily sensation by jumping to the worst possible (and also the least likely) conclusion—that your condition has worsened or signals the onset of a new illness. Once you have a troublesome illness, particularly one for which doctors can't find a very satisfactory diagnosis, it's hard not to misattribute benign bodily sensations and trivial symptoms to that illness. So you jump to the (faulty) conclusion that your disorder is worsening or spreading or progressing.

Before you started having the symptom that bothers you, you may have chalked up these sorts of benign irritants (like headaches or rashes) to aging or too little sleep or poor diet or stress. But now that you're suffering, you conclude that they're related to the illness when in fact they're not—they're just part of the normal wear and tear of life.

When you begin to catastrophize, it is important to take a step back, talk yourself down, take a deep breath, count to ten, and think more logically and rationally about the situation. Have you ever had the same symptom in the past, when it turned out to be nothing serious? Have you ever had the same symptom before and found that it went away on its own? Can you think of less threatening explanations for the symptom than a worsening of your illness? Which of these explanations are actually most likely? If a friend told you the same story, what would you suspect was the cause of his or her symptom? We can often think more calmly and more rationally about someone else's health than our own, especially in an anxious situation.

Depression often lightens when you take action or control of a situation. Do something that makes you feel good about yourself. Get up, shower, and get dressed even if you don't feel like it. Exercise, go for a walk, and have a structured enjoyable activity to look forward to every day. Plan ahead and make out a daily schedule for the next week of things you would normally do (like eating regular meals, getting your hair done), and of activities that were pleasurable before you became depressed (like listening to music, rearranging the furniture, going out to your favorite spot to watch the sunset). Then stick to your schedule each day, whether you feel like it or not. Initially, it may feel as if you're just going through the motions, but eventually they will become pleasurable again. Challenge negative thoughts; reach out and talk to a friend about problems. Volunteer or get involved with others in a common project. Since depressed people are too self-critical and have too negative an opinion of themselves, it's important to think positive and kind thoughts about yourself. When you recognize a self-punishing, negative thought about yourself, deliberately replace it with a kinder, more positive thought. Try to talk to yourself in the same compassionate way you would to a friend who had the same problem.

Many people find it easy to help and take care of others, but they feel guilty or selfish about taking care of themselves. Depression tends to exaggerate this attitude. Laura Calloway began to feel seriously depressed just one month after having her first child. Despite the fact that she cried all the time and ate next to nothing, it was only when she could no longer breastfeed her son, due to her own dehydration, that she could be convinced to get help. For the first several weeks of her treatment, only the reminder that she would be a better mother to her son if she were feeling better could convince her to continue. At the time, she did not care about her own health.

It boosts mood to deliberately take more time to care for yourself in healthy ways. Being selfish about your health and happiness is not a character flaw—it is essential to feeling your best. And remember, if you feel better, you'll be more able to care for your family and friends and those who rely on you. Giving to yourself means you have more to give to everyone else.

As we discussed earlier, being depressed makes us dwell on negative thoughts and events and makes us appraise situations in a pessimistic light. It's natural to be depressed about being sick, but it may be getting you down more than necessary. If so, it's only making your symptoms and your suffering even worse. Try to think through exactly what it is about your illness that is most upsetting.

Some people are most upset by the activity limitations that their illness and their symptoms impose on them; for others, the most depressing thing about being sick is that it makes them feel powerless and not in control of their lives; some people feel less lovable when they're sick, and that's what upsets them most about it; others feel that illness is a punishment they deserve for something they feel guilty about.

Once you have a clearer understanding of exactly what it is about being ill that is most upsetting and depressing, you can try to do something about it. If your symptoms have made you curtail your activities, begin exploring other activities you could substitute for those you've had to give up. If you can no longer go running for exercise, could you take up golf or bike riding? If you can't travel as much as you used to, can you get involved in something closer to home, like a book group?

If you are feeling powerless and out of control, begin figuring out what aspects of your life you do have control over and make sure you're doing those things. If you feel less lovable and less valuable and worthwhile as a person because you're sick, examine carefully how realistic that is; is it really true—if the roles were reversed, would you love your child or your spouse less because he or she was sick? If you feel as if you're being punished, that in some way you deserve what has happened to you, begin focusing on the things about you that you feel are deserving and good, like your skill at decorating the house or your ability to teach your grandchild to read. If you're a religious person, it may help to speak with your clergy about the things you think you're guilty of and about whether illness really is a punishment from God.

Even with the numerous resources online and in the bookstore, sometimes anxiety and depression are too severe to conquer on your own. There are now several successful treatments available for both conditions; some include medication and some do not. If the anxiety and depression are so severe that you feel life is no longer worth living or you think about ending your life, see your doctor right away.

Tony's buddy from Ladder 32 comes to visit Tony at home. His friend talks about his experience with the burns and his recovery. Tony opens up a little, too, about his symptoms, his idea that he is physically ill, and about his feelings that he is no good to his family. His friend admits that he was very depressed after being burned, and that he felt a lot of the same things. What helped him was to get back to his old routines and to focus on activities that made him feel good. He invites Tony to go for a jog with him the next day, as long as Tony "takes it easy" on him and doesn't go too fast.

When Tony gets up at the early hour he used to and puts on his running shoes, he starts to feel better. He realizes just how much he has been dwelling on negative things and his feelings of being so weak. After the run, Tony decides to do something healthy that makes him feel good every time he starts to focus on being depressed or ill.

Dealing with anger can be tricky, but the most important first step is to acknowledge it for what it is. There are so many societal strictures against being angry that some people have a hard time recognizing irritability and a nasty mood as true anger.

Once you've recognized your anger, you can start to figure out the automatic thoughts behind intense angry feelings—thoughts such as "It's so unfair," "My husband is such a jerk," or "I can't take ONE MORE MINUTE of this." These thoughts can lead to acting in unhelpful ways: picking a fight with your spouse; leaving an important meeting or situation before the work is done; or even behaving in a destructive way, such as throwing things or being physically violent. If you get used to tracking your angry feelings and thoughts and make some plans ahead of time, you can channel your outrage into more productive behaviors, like organizing a neighborhood watch or starting an exercise program. You've probably heard the old adage, "Don't get mad, get even." Some of the exercises at the end of the chapter are specifically geared toward getting a better understanding of and redirecting anger.

If someone is doing something that irritates you, it's often best to speak up about it early on, before they've done it so many times that you're really furious and finally blow your stack and overreact. Because the irritant seems unimportant at first, you may tend to bite your tongue, say nothing, and suppress your annoyance. But since you haven't let others know about your feelings, they don't change what they're doing and they keep irritating you unknowingly. Eventually you become so irate that you can no longer contain it, and you blow up inappropriately. You feel foolish for "losing it," and the other person is so shocked and hurt by your response that they just dismiss your complaint as crazy.

Once you are not as angry, you will notice changes in your physical symptoms—changes connected to lower blood pressure, less gastrointestinal distress, and a greater sense of contentment. Hostility, by activating the fight-or-flight response of the nervous and endocrine systems, can worsen many health problems, including heart disease and even wound healing.

In the case of dangerous acting out, including violence to yourself or others, it is vital to seek professional help. Classes on anger management are available in almost any midsize or larger community. Some are even offered for free. Individual treatment, such as therapy, can also be lifesaving if you have uncontrolled, violent anger.

Once Tony began to feel better about himself, he recognized he was being too sensitive to criticism from his wife. In a gentle way, when they were not arguing, he let her know what kinds of comments really annoyed him, and he apologized for his overreactions in the past. Once the lines of communication were open again between Tony and his wife, he found he became much less angry.

Exercises

1. Understand the connection between facial expression and mood.

Raise your eyebrows and show your teeth. Hold this expression for twenty seconds. What kinds of thoughts enter your mind (besides thoughts about looking silly)? How are you feeling?

Relax, then bring your eyebrows together and clench your jaws. For extra effect, clench your fists as well. What are you thinking and feeling now?

As you might have guessed, the first expression signals a smile, the second signals anger. When we maintain these expressions for a while, our body actually goes through changes associated with the emotion. Sometimes simply smiling and standing up straight can alleviate feelings of sadness, even if we don't feel like smiling.

Of course, changing facial expression and posture can't solve the real-world problems that can lead to emotional discomforts. Our aim is to do whatever we can to keep moods from intensifying physical symptoms.

2. Know your anxiety and depression zappers.

Make a list of things you do that relax you. Then make a list of things that make you feel good about yourself. Whenever you feel anxious or blue, take out the lists and start from the top!

3. Track your automatic thoughts.

Do you have automatic negative thoughts that are making you feel more depressed or anxious on a regular basis? In previous chapters, you paid special attention to thoughts related to your symptoms. Now see if you have thoughts related to moods. They tend to take familiar forms, such as, "I am a loser"; "I'll never be able to accomplish anything"; or "This is too much for me." You know they are automatic, because they play in your head whenever you face a stressful or difficult situation.

4. Undo negative thinking.

Write down your automatic negative thoughts on one side of a piece of paper. On the other side, write down a countering thought. When you catch yourself thinking the negative automatic thought, immediately use your rehearsed countering thought.

Automatic Thought	Countering Thought
"I'm a loser."	"That's my depression talking. I've done plenty of good things with my life."
"My husband/wife never understands."	"I can find a way to make my husband/wife understand what is going on with me."
"I can never do anything right."	"I arranged a retirement party for my dad, and everyone had a good time."

5. Weigh in on anger.

The first step to letting go of maladaptive anger is to figure out where anger is helpful and harmful in your life.

Make two lists side by side. In the left column, write advantages to being angry. Some advantages could be that it feels good to shout and get the feelings out, or that there is some satisfaction in revenge, or letting someone know that you are no pushover. Now, in the right-hand column, write the disadvantages of being angry. Some common answers include feeling guilty about hurting someone's feelings with an angry outburst or foolish that you lost control of yourself.

Look at your left-hand column, and try to figure out ways to reap the advantages of anger without getting dragged down by the disadvantages. How can you let your boss know you are no pushover without an angry outburst? How can you get your feelings out about being unfairly stuck with chronic pain or other symptoms without alienating your loved ones by acting out in maladaptive ways?

6. Take control of your anger.

If angry outbursts get you in trouble or raise your blood pressure, it's time to take control of your anger. One way to do this is to "rehearse" a situation that makes you angry ahead of time. Make a list of situations that really anger you, and put them in order of how much they bother you, from least bothersome (such as the car in front of you not moving fast enough at a green light) at the top to most bothersome (for example, seeing a group of teenagers throwing rocks at a stray dog) at the bottom. Now start at the top of the list, with the mildest situation. Imagine going through that situation, and picture how you will keep control over your anger. In the situation with the car at the green light, you might try to count to ten or turn up the radio to distract you. Keep going down the list until you have figured out a way to defuse your anger in each situation.

7. Use a mood chart: take this week to track how your moods affect your symptoms.

Date/Time	Mood	Body Sensation	Intervention	Result
May 16, 7:30 a.m.	Depressed—I just couldn't get out of bed this morning.	My stomach ached. Do I have an ulcer?	Got up, got dressed, ate breakfast.	Knot in stomach went away—my mood is lighter, too.
May 18, 10 p.m.	Anxious—saw on the news that the stock market isn't going well.	My migraine headache might be coming back.	Turned off the news, started to read a book I really love.	That migraine headache never came on.

8. Reap the benefits of expressive writing.

Recently, interest has grown in expressive writing as a way of coping with emotional distress that is detrimental to health.[2]

In studies of rheumatoid arthritis and asthma, patients who are asked to write repeatedly about the most emotionally disturbing experience of their lives report beneficial effects on their physical and psychological symptoms.[3] It is still not known whether this emotionally expressive writing actually affects the body's physiology and the severity of disease, but it is clear that it improves symptoms.

In these studies, patients are instructed to write or to speak into a tape recorder about the most distressing trauma they've experienced in their lives, and to make those narratives as vivid as possible by including their deepest emotions and thoughts, and their bodily sensations. They are asked to do this for about twenty minutes per day for four or five days. While they often report increases in emotional distress immediately after the expressive writing, several months later, when compared to people who wrote about neutral topics that were not stressful, they report they are better in several ways: they feel better physically and have fewer symptoms; they report less psychological and emotional distress; and they are able to function better. They even make fewer visits to the doctor and have fewer absences from work.[4]

So, if you feel ready, set aside twenty minutes a day for the next four or five days. (The expressive writing can take the place of your relaxation practice for this week, if you like.) Take out a composition notebook or open up the word processor and give expressive writing a try. Remember to use all your senses, and try to use vivid words to describe what you've been feeling.

* * *

You've now learned a lot about how certain emotions and moods affect physical symptoms. You've also figured out different ways to alleviate depression, dissipate anxiety, and redirect maladaptive anger. By going to the source and easing these problems with mood, you've decreased the physical symptoms from anxiety (such as stomach churning and lower tolerance for pain), from depression (such as feeling exhausted), and from anger (including having higher blood pressure). Monitoring moods, understanding how they affect symptoms, and doing as much as you can to alleviate depression and anxiety and redirecting anger can decrease your preoccupation with and disability from chronic medical symptoms.

CHAPTER EIGHT

Week 6—Lessons in Coping Well

You have completed the first five weeks of the program. By now, you have a good handle on all sorts of reasons your symptoms get better or worse. We've studied the attention and focus you give your symptoms and how your thinking changes how you feel. We've also learned how different circumstances—whether stressful situations or interpersonal relationships, the ways you behave, and your moods—all affect your symptoms.

This week, our focus will be on pulling together everything you have learned to continue to cope successfully with your symptoms. First, we will give some attention to what makes someone good at coping and enables him or her to live more comfortably despite illness.

Coping is problem-solving behavior that is designed to reduce, manage, or tolerate stressful events that we feel are threatening to overwhelm us. People who are especially good at coping are flexible and very open to suggestion. They are able to retain their optimism and keep up their morale despite setbacks. They keep focused on the immediate problem at hand before worrying about more remote or less likely problems. For example, they find ways to get to the supermarket and bring in the groceries from the car despite back pain, rather than dwelling on how bad the pain might become after another year like this one.

Less successful copers, on the other hand, tend to maintain a more rigid outlook and find it harder to compromise and to seek help. They tend to resist other people's suggestions. It is difficult for them to prioritize their problems and their goals, so they spend a lot of time worrying about less important and less likely problems.

The best way to understand good coping is to pay attention to and learn from those who do it well. We'll reflect on the strategies and techniques they use in minimizing their symptoms—ignoring, overcoming, and compensating for them. We will share the stories of one individual who is naturally good at coping, and several others who have learned to cope exceptionally well with the help of our six-week program.

Shane Ridgely

Shane is a fifty-seven-year-old former real estate lawyer and Little League coach who underwent chemotherapy for a particularly malignant form of cancer ten years ago. Although the cancer has not recurred, Shane has had to cope with chronic symptoms and an inexorable series of medical setbacks since then. These have forced him to progressively give up many activities that he had enjoyed and had meant a great deal to him. As he himself put it, "My life has been nibbled away."

First, as a side effect of his successful chemotherapy, Shane developed a blood-clotting problem. This problem resulted in three small strokes that have made it impossible for him to drive a car. The chemotherapy also caused chronic heart and kidney problems, and these have forced him to adopt a very strict diet. The worst part of this diet is that he has had to stop eating hot peppers, which were his favorite food and something he took great joy growing in his own vegetable garden each summer.

The most disturbing of all his symptoms has been chronic fatigue. Shane was so exhausted after treatment that he couldn't continue working and had to retire prematurely. He also had to give up coaching his beloved Little League team.

Shane has certainly had periods of demoralization and dependency over the last ten years, but overall he has managed to maintain a positive outlook and to find ways of coping with his symptoms that allow him to replace his former activities and gratifications with new ones. When he could no longer supervise the junior partners in his firm, he took up tutoring a small number of adults in English as a second language. Though he missed the excitement of the law firm, he found tutoring offered him the chance to get to know individual students better, and he has enjoyed this closer contact.

Shane now goes regularly to minor-league baseball games as a spectator rather than as a coach. He has found he can remain personally involved by closely following the careers of some of the players he formerly coached. As an interested spectator, he does miss the excitement of coaching, but he doesn't miss the pressures that came with being in charge of the Little Leaguers and the tensions of dealing with their parents.

He was surprised to find that his fatigue and poor exercise tolerance have helped him in one respect. When he wanted to build a new garage, Shane asked his son Billy for help. In the past, Shane would have done it himself, but now he was able to spend several months growing closer to his son, offering his knowledge and guidance while Billy provided much of the labor.

Psychologically, Shane has come to accept his chronic symptoms. "There's no point in wishing for things that are not possible," he notes. He remembers being told at the time of his diagnosis that he was unlikely to survive for much more than six months, so he feels fortunate to have lived this long. "All of the life I've had since then has been a gift."

It is this combination of perspective and ingenuity, flexibility, and resourcefulness in adjusting to his progressive physical limitations that has stood Shane in such good stead. He learned to substitute one form of tutoring for another, to get pleasure from giving his hot peppers away to appreciative neighbors instead of eating them himself, and to allow his physical limitations to help him get closer to his son.

Ruth Gutman

The first symptom Ruth Gutman noticed was a pins-and-needles sensation that came and went in her hands and fingertips. A few months later, her gait became unsteady and she sometimes felt dizzy. Later on, she noticed occasional blurring of her vision. At that point she was diagnosed with multiple sclerosis, but then her condition stabilized and showed no neurological signs of worsening.

Although her symptoms did not get worse, Ruth found it harder and harder to live with them. She thought constantly about her illness, tormenting herself with what might happen decades in the future. Her worst nightmare was becoming a burden and a drain on her family. She was haunted by the image of her husband, Ben, having to push her everywhere in a wheelchair while her medical and drug bills drained the family finances. She just couldn't seem to get that vision out of her head.

The more worried she became, the more closely she monitored her symptoms, looking for any sign that they were progressing. She wondered if her walk was becoming clumsier, or if others noticed a tremor in her hands. She became extremely self-conscious, which in itself made her movements more stilted and awkward, further terrifying her.

Her neurologist repeatedly assured her that there was no evidence of any disease progression, and that her condition might remain stable indefinitely. However, she felt compelled to learn as much as she could about multiple sclerosis on the Internet. There she encountered numerous sites with horrifying, personal stories of catastrophic illnesses that left sufferers paralyzed, blind, and incontinent. All of this only fueled her anxiety, amplified her symptoms, and further preoccupied her.

Ruth was eventually referred to our six-week program for coping with chronic symptoms. Using the program, Ruth was able to put her illness in perspective and reverse the spiral she had gotten into. Seeing how her Internet searches were actually making her feel worse, Ruth was able to progressively cut back the time devoted to this and then to substitute searches about collecting pottery, her longstanding hobby. As she understood how her self-consciousness, rather than advancing multiple sclerosis, was making her movements more awkward and clumsy, she was able to relax a bit and notice that the symptoms seemed less prominent.

Her counselor helped her to see how anxiety was making her think irrationally, how she was catastrophizing and worrying about the most horrific possible outcomes and thinking decades in the future, rather than focusing on the more likely outcomes and the near future. They agreed on a treatment plan for anxiety that included relaxation response training and a mild tranquilizer for a few months.

As her anxiety diminished, she noticed the symptoms less often and they seemed less intrusive and less bothersome. Finally, the therapist encouraged her to discuss her illness fully with her husband, including telling him her fears of ultimately becoming dependent on him and a burden to him. She hadn't found Ben to be very supportive or reassuring in the past, but it turned out that this was because he had no idea what was bothering her. He couldn't really respond or be helpful when he had no insight into what was on her mind. As he later put it, "Trying to reassure Ruth back then was like telling a crying, sleepless child not to fear the monster under the bed, when what he actually fears is the strange noise outside his window." Once Ben understood Ruth's fears of dependence on him, they were able to discuss and allay some of her concerns.

Luis Navarro

Luis Navarro is a seventy-year-old retired restaurant owner who developed episodes of squeezing chest pain five years ago. He went to his doctor and was found to have significant blockage of the coronary arteries. Since then, Luis's pain has been a source of significant disability and worry to him. He used to be a daily runner, and he trained with weights several times a week. When he was in his sixties, people often mistook him for someone in his forties or fifties. After his diagnosis though, he stopped exercising.

He also sold his restaurant and retired, worrying that the stress of the job might worsen his heart disease. Before his illness, he and his wife loved to travel all over the world. After his chest pain began, he limited his travel for fear that his condition might worsen while he was far from home and from his doctors. He even stopped having intimate relations with his wife, afraid that the excitement could cause deadly stress on his heart.

Luis gradually became excessively concerned about his symptoms and preoccupied with his illness. He followed an extremely stringent, low-fat diet; scrupulously monitored his blood pressure six times a day and averaged the readings; and collected huge files of clippings about heart disease from newspapers, magazines, and newsletters. He saw several different cardiologists regularly, and visited them armed with sophisticated and specific questions, such as the benefits of drinking grape juice, the value of the test for C-reactive protein, and the details of President Clinton's coronary artery bypass surgery.

Luis has had several life events that have made him more vulnerable to anxiety about his heart than most other patients: his own father died suddenly at the age of forty-eight of a heart rhythm disturbance, and two of his brothers have had serious heart problems. As a result, he has long been worried about heart disease and has even thought that he was destined to die prematurely of a heart attack.

Luis was eventually referred by his doctor to the six-week program for coping with symptoms because he felt Luis had become excessively anxious about his heart. Over the course of a half-dozen counseling sessions, Luis was helped to identify his personal strengths and use them to deal with his symptoms more adaptively. First, he came to see that he had too much time on his hands and really missed his work. "If I were busier," he said, "I don't think I'd spend so much time on my health." He turned to some pet projects he had never had the time to work on before. During his time as a restaurant owner, Luis had invented several gadgets that worked well in his commercial kitchen, streamlining cooking times and service. Now he presented a large restaurant chain with his inventions, and was offered a part-time job consulting for them.

Luis asked one of his brothers, a lawyer, to help him with legal advice about patenting his gadgets. As the commercial potential for his ideas emerged, Luis spent a lot of time with his brother. It became a chance to heal some old rifts that had developed between the two of them. Luis became more preoccupied with whether he could interest the chain in introducing his invention rather than in whether his blood pressure was higher or lower than it had been the day before. And he certainly found his new preoccupation more enjoyable and more rewarding than his former one.

Luis also came to realize that some of what he was doing to monitor his condition and treat himself was amplifying his symptoms and leading to increased health-related anxiety. When surfing the Internet in hopes of discovering reassuring information about new therapies for heart disease, he almost always ended up more frightened by what he came across. Likewise, his habit of asking his various doctors to tell him with absolute certainty that his heart disease was not advancing resulted in more anxiety, because while they told him they were sure that was the case, they admitted they could never be 100 percent certain. He was also helped to see that repeatedly checking his blood pressure and counting how many steps he could climb before becoming short of breath each day was only amplifying his symptoms and increasing his preoccupation with his heart. Having discovered the paradoxical consequences of his behaviors, he was able to begin curtailing them. As he did this, Luis found that the symptoms themselves became less problematic. At the last of his counseling sessions, Luis announced triumphantly that he had decided to throw out all of the old clipping files he had collected on heart disease.

Finally, Luis was encouraged by his counselor to have a frank talk with his primary care physician about what they were trying to accomplish with his medical management and how they could best work together. Luis expressed his misgivings and reservations about his medical care—in particular, that seeing so many different doctors had left him confused by their sometimes slightly contradictory or conflicting messages. Luis and his physician agreed on a schedule of regular visits every eight weeks, regardless of how Luis was feeling. At these appointments, they would plan Luis's medication regimen and self-treatment program for the next eight weeks and would not make any changes in the plan in between the regularly scheduled appointments (unless, of course, his medical situation changed drastically). This had the effect of easing the pressure Luis felt to stay on top of his symptoms minute by minute and to continually update himself on the latest medical information, since these would no longer prompt any change in his treatment until the next doctor visit. For example, since he won't change his consumption of grape juice or his aspirin dose between appointments, he doesn't need to look on the Internet or watch all the morning news shows every day in order to catch the latest thinking about them.

After several years of not doing well, Luis now exemplifies some of the keys to good coping. He was able to find a passion that captured his interest and his time. He also managed to use this new activity as a way to enrich his family life by getting closer to his brother. He discovered that while he could not stop his chest pain from occurring, he could change the way he responded to it, and this in turn helped make the symptom less disturbing and disabling. Finally, in collaboration with his doctor, he learned to arrange his medical care in such a way that it became more a source of reassurance and less a source of alarm and anxiety.

Dr. Marissa Stokes

Marissa Stokes is a fifty-eight-year-old dentist who sustained a nerve injury in her right hand that left it weak and clumsy. Although she regained a good deal of function in her hand, she never regained the high degree of fine-motor coordination that dentistry requires. This left her emotionally crushed and changed her life profoundly. While she learned, with practice, to perform many daily tasks, she was still unable to tie her shoes, shuffle a deck of cards (bridge with her friends was a longtime passion), or even pick out the right change at the store.

Most importantly, she had to stop practicing dentistry. As she said, "My area of expertise used to be doing complicated dental restorations; now my area of expertise is emptying out the dishwasher." She had a strong, authoritative nature, and didn't like the changes resulting from her premature retirement. "In my own private office, I used to be the one giving the orders; now I seem to be the one taking them."

Marissa especially hated the reversal of roles in her life—she went from being a health care professional to being the patient. Instead of wearing a white coat and treating patients, she now found herself sitting in waiting rooms and having other professionals in white coats treat her. This made her feel humiliated and ashamed.

With the loss of her profession, she felt diminished as a person, less respected and less important. She began to argue with her husband and became more touchy. She was prone to feeling that others were treating her disrespectfully, from the checker at the grocery store to her nieces and nephews who visited for Christmas. She felt as if she were being dismissed, that her opinions were disregarded. She was frequently irritated with salespeople and gas station attendants, sometimes even getting into arguments with them. While her husband continued to work, she felt the long days bitterly, and began to sense that even he was ignoring her, and their fights worsened.

Not surprisingly, Marissa became demoralized and depressed. Her injury damaged her self-image, robbing her of what she most valued about herself—her identity as an esteemed professional, and her independence. She especially resented losing that sense of autonomy that came from earning a salary and supporting herself financially.

At several times in her life, Marissa had narrowly escaped serious injury and even death—it almost seemed as if fate had intervened each time. Once, she had been saved from a mugging late at night purely through luck, as a policeman happened to be driving by at the time. On another occasion, soon after she began her dental career in the army, she escaped a fatal explosion at the army base where she worked. She had always felt that her good luck meant that she was supposed to survive, that God had spared her life because she had been put on earth to practice her profession and to help others. She could not make sense of this new illness that prevented her from fulfilling her purpose in life. What was her mission now? She wondered if her illness were some sort of punishment for something she might have done. She was confused and dismayed. Without her profession, her life seemed to have little meaning.

Her husband begged her to get help, and Marissa decided to try the six-week program to help her to learn more about how her illness experiences, attitudes, and behaviors were impairing the quality of her life.

As Marissa began learning to cope with her symptoms, her personal strengths emerged. She had always enjoyed yoga, but now took it up more seriously as a successful distraction from her symptoms. Though she still couldn't control her hand, yoga helped her regain the experience of being able to control her body and her movements. Her improving technique and physical fitness made her feel less diminished, damaged, and disabled.

She also learned to think more creatively about her profession. She had been boxed in by the idea that she was useless without her right hand. But just because she couldn't practice dentistry didn't mean she was finished as a dentist. She took on a teaching job at the local dental school and became a consultant to the training program there. With time, she began to relish her role as a teacher and mentor, seeing it as a way in which her skills and experience would live on in the skillful hands of her trainees.

Marissa discovered how her attitudes and behaviors had kept her feeling miserable. As she felt less diminished and demeaned, she stopped waiting for shop clerks and relatives to be disrespectful, and instead disarmed surly checkout personnel with a smile. When her niece was fresh, she relied on her old authoritative manner to direct the child to treat her with respect instead of sulking and complaining. She took control of situations that she could, and learned to let go those that she could not change.

She began to track her moods and see how they made her more self-conscious of the clumsiness in her hand and made her think more negatively about her husband. She learned to tell him that she wasn't in the mood for arguing or sarcasm, and did her part in avoiding petty arguments. She took up the hobby of digital photography and went on day trips with her husband to photograph scenes around their neighborhood in different seasons and weather.

In successfully coming to terms with a serious, chronic symptom, Marissa demonstrated some valuable personal qualities and highly adaptive strategies. She dealt with a deficit by developing a compensatory strength—she compensated for weakness and loss of coordination in her hand by getting generally stronger and more coordinated through yoga. She discovered a way of exercising her

professional skill through others, by teaching them her
techniques and knowledge, so that her work was carried
on through their hands. Finally, now that she had free
time, she turned more to her family and grew closer to
her husband. In short, Marissa made lemons into lemonade and avoided making mountains out of molehills.[1]

Ongoing Practice

Shane, Ruth, Luis, and Marissa all went through
major life changes as the result of chronic medical symptoms. While Shane was naturally good at adapting to his
new life, Ruth, Luis, and Marissa struggled with their illnesses for a long time before they learned new ways to
cope and be fulfilled despite limitations. At the end of
these six weeks, you will have gained a lot of wisdom
about what particular strategies and situations help you
feel better and cope with your symptoms. Now your task
is to discover the most useful exercises and ways of thinking you have learned, and to create a plan to keep practicing successful coping even after you close this book.

Exercises

FIND THE SUCCESSFUL COPING SKILLS WITHIN YOU

1. Do you have anything in common with Shane, Ruth,
Luis, or Marissa? Think of ways you can be more flexible
in your expectations for yourself, taking into account the
realistic limitations of your symptoms. Marissa found
she could be fulfilled by teaching her skills and experience to others, for example, and Luis consulted in the
restaurant business instead of running the business

himself. Is there a way you can adjust to your symptoms but still continue to pursue the essence of what you love?

2. Did your symptoms change your life plans in any way? Even though your illness is unwelcome, have there been any advantages to your life course being changed? How can you make lemonade from lemons? Perhaps fatigue makes it impossible to work a forty-hour-a-week job, but how can you use your time to become more fulfilled as a person? Could you spend more time with loved ones, working on a pet project, volunteering, or pursuing hobbies you never had time for before?

3. How have your symptoms changed your relationships with your friends and family? Have any relationships actually improved? Why? Have any become worse? In what ways? Are there ways to change your roles in these relationships to make them better?

DISTILL THE MOST USEFUL EXERCISES FOR YOUR STRENGTHS, LIMITATIONS, AND PERSONALITY FROM THE SIX-WEEK PROGRAM

1. Go back through your exercise workbook. Were there any particular exercises that were very helpful for you? What exactly made that particular exercise useful? Did it help your symptom improve physically? Did it change your outlook in other ways?

2. In your review of your workbook, you probably found some exercises that you either skipped or felt were not useful to you at all. Why were they not helpful? For example, meditation is not everyone's "cup of tea." Did any of the exercises make your symptoms worse (for example,

sometimes breathing exercises can make anxious people feel more lightheaded)? What did you learn about yourself and your symptoms from the exercises that didn't work for you? It is important to understand that some suggestions and techniques won't work for you, and you don't need to spend more time and energy trying to make them work. And don't beat yourself up over it. It is just as important to recognize strategies that, for whatever reason, simply aren't right for you as it is to identify and work on the things that are helpful.

3. What was the most surprising part of the last five weeks? Did you discover that your symptoms get suddenly worse in the presence of someone you know, or that you were using your symptoms to get out of activities you don't like to do? Do you think that letting others know how much your symptoms bothered you was sometimes a way of eliciting special consideration or support that you couldn't have gotten otherwise? Did you find better ways to express your likes and dislikes than through feeling physically ill?

4. What part of your symptoms and how they feel has not changed at all? Do your symptoms feel better, or has your attitude about your symptoms changed in positive ways, so that your life is starting to be better? Does it matter as much if there may be no cure or no definitive medical explanation for your pains and symptoms if you can improve your life despite them?

5. The following worksheet combines all the areas we focused on these last five weeks. Using the examples as a guide, try to use all the different modalities listed to understand and change something about your symptom or the way you deal with it. Feel free to go back to previous chapters to see which strategies worked for you.

Symptom	Chest pain
Attention	I was waiting for my son to come home from his late-night date—the quiet of the house made me notice my pain more. I used distraction by turning on my favorite music to keep my mind off the pain.
Thoughts	As usual, I thought: "Here it is again. Eventually I'm going to get a heart attack just like my father." I noticed my automatic thought and immediately thought of a counter— "My doctor told me this pain is not from heart disease. Right now my heart is healthy."
Behaviors	In the past when my chest hurt, I would call my son and ask him to pick up some groceries for me. Then I felt guilty about cutting his evening short. Now I'm going to try shopping at times when the store and the parking lot are less crowded, rather than relying on someone else.
Circumstances	My pain always seems to get worse when I am worrying about my son, or when I hear about bad things on the news. I've decided to watch a game show at 6:30 instead of the evening news. That's thirty minutes a day now I don't feel so bad!
Moods	For a while, I was getting very depressed about my limitations. Then I noticed that my depressed mood made my pain worse! Now I try to think about the things I can do, such as gardening, rather than the things I can't.
Coping	I realize now that I have a lot of strategies and ways of dealing with my pain I never did before.

6. In the first exercise in this section, you listed several strategies and activities that were most helpful for you. Now make a schedule or a weekly calendar to continue making these a part of your day. On the facing page is one example, using meditation and relaxation as the useful activity you want to continue. Feel free to make your own calendar with a different activity, such as exercise, or even combining and trading off activities. For example, on Monday, distract yourself by doing something fun (seeing a movie, making dessert). On Tuesday, be sure to exercise. On every other day, do ten minutes of mindful meditation. Make the schedule something

Feet numb from diabetes
My numb feet are making me crazy! I tried a meditation exercise. Something about being in the moment and breathing through the sensation helps me tolerate the numb feeling better.
"I'm going to lose my feet to diabetes." Counter—"I can watch my diet and take my medication, and that will help me keep my feet and preserve the sensation that I have left."
I used to sit and mope about my feet, and sitting still only made everything worse. I was able to get an orthopedic shoe that is safe for me to walk in—so today I took a walk instead of sitting around.
I notice my feet more when my wife wants me to help out around the house. When I recognized that fact, somehow my feet seemed to bug me less! I try to do the chores I don't mind so much, and that helps too.
I was really irritable when my feet went numb, and I kept snapping at everyone around me. I made a list of what makes me angry and why for the exercises in the moods chapter. Now I feel more prepared when irritation strikes.
I thought my diabetes would ruin my life. It certainly has changed it. I haven't figured everything out yet, but I feel better, even though my feet are still numb. I can still do many of the things I enjoy. Life is good.

reasonable that you will be able to follow. And most importantly, don't feel guilty if you miss a day—just start again with the next day!

Monday: Twenty minutes sitting meditation—diaphragmatic breathing
Tuesday: Yoga DVD
Wednesday: Twenty minutes sitting meditation—diaphragmatic breathing
Thursday: Progressive muscle relaxation, followed by mindfulness
Friday: Yoga DVD

Saturday: Twenty minutes sitting meditation—diaphragmatic breathing
Sunday: Off!

Congratulations!

You have now completed the six-week program to stop being your symptoms and start being yourself. You have learned a great deal to help you become an expert at coping, and you have a solid plan to continue practicing your coping skills until they become second nature to you.

We all get into cycles of healthy and unhealthy habits. You may find, in the future, that you have fallen back into old ways of thinking and feeling that worsen your symptoms again. In that case, you should start again at the first week and continue all the way through the book. Try to do any exercises you may have skipped the first time, or focus on a different area of the program (more meditation, or a minimal amount of relaxation activity, instead using a distracting, healthy activity such as physical exercise). Each time through you may discover some new coping mechanism or strength within yourself.

The last part of this book is dedicated to extending your practice, learning several different ways to feel your best, including nutrition and exercise guidelines for those with chronic symptoms. By now you have done a lot of hard work and have become an expert on what makes your symptoms feel better or worse. The next two chapters contain just a little extra information to help you continue to feel better and take charge of your symptoms, and the way you live your life.

PART THREE

General Principles for
Living and Coping Well

CHAPTER NINE

Living Well Through Nutrition and Exercise

No book about coping with symptoms is complete without a good look at all the basic ways to help improve health, regulate mood, and lessen pain. Two of the most important contributors to how you feel are what you eat and how you move. What you eat is the building block for your muscles, organs, and nerves, and has everything to do with your energy levels throughout the day. How you move affects not only your strength, balance, and flexibility, but if done properly can release all sorts of natural painkillers and relaxation molecules in your body.

For people suffering with chronic symptoms, proper nutrition and reasonable exercise can be a great way to improve health and vitality without side effects or doctor's visits. Given that we've spent the last six chapters giving you lots of work to do with paper, pencil, planning, thinking, and relaxation, the last thing we want to do is add any complications to your life. So this chapter is designed to be a basic primer, giving general guidelines to the best sorts of nutrients and exercise for people often left less mobile with chronic pain and other ongoing symptoms.

Pete Frederick was a married father of two children. At age thirty-five, he wasn't nearly as fit or active as he'd been back in college. Nights spent eating chips and drinking beer in front of the television left its mark on his steadily expanding belly. He didn't have the time to exercise; with the mortgage and his first kid going off to college in only four years, he needed to work all he could. He relieved his stress by smoking a pack a day. His time on the front porch with his cigarette was the only alone time he got all day.

His diet during the day wasn't much better than his TV food at night. He would usually eat a donut or pastry for breakfast, if he managed to eat at all. At lunchtime, he'd go to a fast food drive-through, or hit the vending machine for cookies and chips. He drank soda throughout the day at work, and in the evening, his busy working wife would bring home more fast food for the family, or order a pizza.

About a month after his thirty-fifth birthday, he started to notice stomach pains. Almost every day he had a dull ache in his abdomen. The pain intensified to cramps, and one day it was so bad he had to call in sick to work. He decided to go to the doctor.

Like many younger men, Pete hadn't made many trips to the doctor. The nurse took his vital signs and clucked her teeth when she checked his blood pressure. She told him it was too high, and ordered him to relax. He tried some deep breaths, but as soon as the cuff went around his arm for a second try, he started to tense up again. The repeat reading was even higher.

Once he saw the doctor, he explained what his stomach pain felt like. Sometimes burning, but often more of a dull ache that he experienced most of the time. The doctor ordered some lab tests and wrote him a couple of prescriptions for his stomach. She warned him to stop smoking, and told him to come back in two weeks. If his blood pressure wasn't any better, he would have to go on medication.

Months passed, and he was put on different medicine for

his stomach and started new pills for his blood pressure. The pain continued, and so did the medical tests, from swallowing barium to getting scoped down his throat. His doctor ordered him to change his diet and once again warned him about the dangers of smoking when he had such high blood pressure.

Pete didn't change his diet, and the pain was so stressful for him, he couldn't even imagine quitting smoking. Cookies and cake made him feel good right after he ate them. He didn't enjoy much in his life, so the thought of changing his diet over to "rabbit food" seemed terrible.

About six months after his pain started, he ran into his friend Roy at a neighborhood holiday party. Roy and he had gone to college together, and had spent many nights drinking beer and watching football. The last time he saw Roy, his friend had been topping 250 pounds. He had asthma and carried around inhalers. Now, at the party, Roy looked fantastic. He'd lost the sixty extra pounds and looked fit and healthy.

Roy and Pete started talking. Pete asked him how he lost the weight and what it was like eating rabbit food all the time. Roy laughed and told him it wasn't all rabbit food and it wasn't all that bad—though it did take a commitment to changing his habits. But it was worth it, Roy said. He no longer needed inhalers, and he felt better and happier than he ever had in his life.

Managing Your Mood with Food

These days, it's very easy to get confused about what food is good for you. We've gone from the four food groups to food pyramids to vegetarian, no fat, organic, light, and low carbohydrate. The same confusing media hype about medical problems and symptoms has also been applied to the press about the basic principles of nutrition. Just as every new conflicting medical study is printed with the exciting promise of cures right around the corner, new nutrition studies are trumpeted by the media and every diet guru trying to make a few dollars. Calcium is the key...Go low-glycemic... Bananas are bad—no, bananas are good! Eggs are bad...Eggs aren't so bad after all! There's even a Web site about the evils of puffed wheat. The only piece left out of all this media nutrition wrangling is common sense.

But common sense isn't quite as straightforward as it seems. Some of the principles we may have learned as kids—such as eat three meals a day, clean your plate, and don't snack between meals—have turned out to be the wrong advice too. The good news is the best way to eat for having steady physical and mental energy is easy enough to be listed in five basic rules:

1. Eat small amounts frequently throughout the day, starting with breakfast.

2. Eat unprocessed, natural foods as much as possible.

3. Eat a variety of nutrients in a variety of colors.

4. Avoid saturated fats and trans-fats.

5. Choose the right supplements.

First we will explain the ins and outs of all these commonsense rules, then we will put together a basic meal plan to help you see just how easy it is to follow the rules and still eat great-tasting food. Before you feel overwhelmed by the rules, realize also that each one can be helpful on its own. If you're not ready to dive into a totally new way of eating, try to follow just one of the rules, and you'll be improving your energy and nutrition.

Eat Small Amounts Frequently Throughout the Day, Starting with Breakfast

Somewhere along the way, food became the enemy of health. After all, excessive amounts of food lead to obesity, diabetes, and cancer. Too much of the wrong kinds of food can cause heart disease, fatty liver, and strokes. Food can be the delivery vehicle for food poisoning, *salmonella, E. coli,* and heavy metals such as mercury. But the real truth is that the key to feeling well lies in what we eat. Our bodies are furnaces, and food is the energy. Eating the best food available will keep our bodies humming and our energy levels regular.

The body's energy level has a name: the metabolic rate. Basically, the metabolic rate is the pace at which the body burns fat and food to keep moving and doing all the processes it does to stay alive and healthy. The faster the metabolic rate, the more calories are burned off at any particular moment. The best way to keep the fires of metabolism stoked is to fuel it frequently and regularly,[1] every three hours at least, up to six times a day. This means snacks are good for you, and the easiest way to slow your metabolism to a crawl is to skip meals or fast.

There are numerous clinical studies from various nutrition journals that show eating more often, up to six times a day, speeds up the metabolic rate compared eating three times a day.[2] Why is this? Well, every time we eat, our metabolism flares up to deal with the new fuel load. The more often you eat, the more often you flare up the metabolism. Athletes who eat more often show lower body fat and increased percentages of muscle.[3] People who eat more often eat less total amount of food during the day, because they don't tend to binge, which helps to keep off the extra pounds.

If you suffer from chronic medical symptoms, you will often be under- or overweight. Fatigue or ongoing nausea or pain can greatly affect appetite and the ability to exercise. If you are underweight and have trouble with appetite or eating a lot at a time, it is vital to eat frequently in order to consume enough calories and nutrients for energy and to make sure your body can make immune proteins and keep the heart and other organs healthy. If you aren't eating enough, it can be difficult for you to regulate body temperature or for the heart to have enough energy to keep you going. Small portions are easier to take in, and they keep the metabolic fires burning and energy levels strong. If you are underweight, you have the opposite problem of the majority of Americans, but the same frequent eating pattern will help you feel better and ensure enough vital fuel for your body.

Chronic symptoms can take a lot from your life, and one of the few enjoyments left may be food. Chronic pain and fatigue also can restrict your ability to exercise, making it much more difficult to burn off the weekend BBQ or your daughter's birthday cake. If, like most Americans, you are overweight, you may have tried many of the major diet plans. You might have noticed that all these plans, including Weight Watchers, South Beach, Body for Life, Jenny Craig, and NutriSystem, recommend three meals a day…plus snacks (two or three a day, depending on the plan). The nutritionists who made those plans know the science about how the body processes food. The best way to burn calories and fat is to eat often, so you never get hungry and you don't gorge yourself.

The most important meal of the day is breakfast.[4] Your mother was right—that wisdom hasn't changed through every breakthrough in nutrition over the past fifty years. When we go from sleeping to waking, our body goes from a hibernating, overnight fast to moving and walking and talking—and it needs fresh fuel to do all of these things. Ironically, skipping breakfast will fool your body into thinking it is starving, raising stress hormones and causing it to hold onto fat and burn your muscle as fuel. Since muscle is metabolically active tissue that burns calories while you are sitting on the couch, the more muscle you have, the more you can eat without gaining fat. Eating breakfast and then eating every three hours thereafter sets the stage for vibrant energy, a speedy metabolism, and keeping muscle from being consumed as fuel.

The final piece to emphasize about the first commonsense nutrition rule is the part about small portions. All the extra benefits from eating frequently are small benefits that eventually add up—a few calories saved here and there that slowly become pounds of fat lost. A controlled portion size is very important if you are trying to maintain or lose weight, or all the caloric and metabolic benefits from eating frequently will be erased. Fortunately, if you eat five to six times a day, it is easier not to binge eat.

Eat Unprocessed, Natural Foods as Much as Possible

Of all the five simple nutrition rules, this one is the most obvious, and probably the most well known. Not only does food supply basic energy to our bodies, it also carries with it water, vitamins, and minerals, all of which are important to keep our bones, muscles, nerves, and organs working well. Most highly processed foods have been stripped of nutrients such as fiber and vitamins. To add insult to injury, processed foods tend to be denser in calories, too. That means you can eat larger volumes of food and feel fuller if you eat whole fruits, raw or steamed vegetables, whole-wheat items, brown rice, oatmeal, and lean animal proteins. These kinds of foods "stick to your ribs" and leave you satisfied without stuffing you with too many calories.

For those of you who are overweight and want to lose a few pounds, you have the tricky task of consuming smaller amounts of food but still needing to get enough vitamins and fiber. The best way to do this is to eat foods closer to their natural, unprocessed state. For those of you who are underweight and don't eat enough, it is vital to get enough vitamins and fiber to keep your system going and to make up for the deficiencies you may already have.

Constipation is a major problem for the undernourished and those who are more immobile due to chronic pain and other symptoms. Not only is constipation uncomfortable, it can make you nauseated and not want to eat. Natural, high-fiber foods such as beans and vegetables keep the gastrointestinal system working smoothly. Other foods high in soluble fiber, such as oatmeal and many fruits, keep your heart healthy by lowering your cholesterol.

Eat a Variety of Nutrients in a Variety of Colors

Food comes in two varieties: *micronutrients* and *macronutrients*. Micronutrients are vitamins, minerals, and phytochemicals (the color chemicals found in natural foods, particularly bright vegetables and fruits such as red peppers and blueberries). Eating lots of different kinds of foods gives you access to lots of different vitamins, minerals, and phytochemicals, so you are less likely to have a deficiency of any of them. The phytochemicals are thought to be powerful cancer-fighting compounds.[5]

The proper ratios of macronutrients—that is, protein, carbohydrates, and fats—have been debated endlessly over the past few decades, particularly high carb/low fat versus low carb/high protein. In order for you to have a good understanding of this debate, it is important to know a little bit about what these macronutrients do in the body.

Protein is the "building block" of the body, especially with regard to muscle tissue, skin, bones, and hair, but it also has roles in all sorts of body processes, including immunity against disease and enabling important chemical reactions. In a pinch, protein can also be burned as fuel in combination with fat. Protein comes from both animal and vegetable sources. Animal sources (meat and dairy) and soy are "complete proteins," meaning they have all the varieties of protein you need for a number of metabolic functions. Vegetable sources such as wheat, rice, or beans are "incomplete proteins," but if combined correctly (for example, rice and beans) they can make complete proteins.

In many ways, protein is a dieter's friend. It is difficult to digest, so you burn more calories eating it than you do eating carbohydrates or fats. That means calorie for calorie, you can eat a bit more protein for the same amount of calorie energy that gets digested. Also, if you want to keep all of your muscle when you are trying to take off extra fat, you need to eat protein frequently to prevent the body from scavenging your muscles for nutrients. Protein can also smooth out the process of digestion so you aren't left with the sugar highs and lows that come from eating pure carbohydrates. Eating a bit of protein with every meal can help keep you satisfied and energetic.

Carbohydrates are the major source of clean-burning

fuel for the body. They come in several varieties: mainly, simple sugars (such as table sugar, syrup, honey, corn syrup, dairy sugars, fruit sugars) and complex carbohydrates (such as corn, rice, beans, vegetables, and wheat). Recently, there has been a lot of media attention about a different way to divide up carbohydrates, into "low-glycemic" and "high-glycemic" carbohydrates.

Low-glycemic carbohydrates do not cause as much of a jump in blood sugar, which means they don't cause the highs and lows you might experience after eating a handful of sugar candy. Sugar highs and lows can lead to binge eating and mood swings, not to mention wildly fluctuating energy levels. Eating a combination of foods with every meal, including protein and some fats, will help protect you from those blood-sugar fluctuations. That means high-glycemic carbohydrates may not necessarily cause spikes in blood sugar if you eat them with lower-glycemic carbohydrates, protein, and/or fat.

Perhaps the best way, from a commonsense standpoint, to divide up the carbohydrates is not by simple and complex or high- and low-glycemic, but rather along a scale of natural to processed. More natural carbohydrates would obviously include fruits, vegetables, and honey. These carbohydrates come packed with vitamins and/or healthy fiber. Even though fruits such as bananas and a simple sugar such as honey are high-glycemic carbohydrates, they have other benefits, such as cancer-fighting antioxidants and B vitamins, which make them valuable sources of nutrients for the body. Also in the more natural category would be sweet potatoes, whole wheat, and brown rice. More processed would be refined sugar such as that found in cakes and candy, and refined white flour and white rice.

More processed foods are almost pure energy without extra vitamins or fiber. These more refined carbohydrates have gotten a bad reputation in recent years, but they are fine to eat if you get enough nutrients and fiber in other ways and are able to burn off all the calorie energy they contain. Some of them (such as highly refined sugars) often come with nutrients that are not good for you in anything but small quantities—namely, saturated fats and trans-fats (in cakes, ice cream, and pastry), or the alcohol in beer, wine, and cocktails.

Carbohydrates are a good source of energy for the body, and they also are vital in shuttling protein in and out of muscle cells. Common sense applies for them as for every other nutrient: Eat several different kinds, the more natural the better, in combination with the other macronutrients, fat and protein. Eating carbohydrates in this way gives you a steady source of clean-burning energy to keep you going strong and your moods steady.

The last macronutrient is *fat*. As in the case of carbohydrates, there has been a lot of media attention on fats over the years, and the information overload is enough to confuse even a registered dietician. Fats are vital for the body to work well and be fueled properly. Every cell in the body is made up of some fat, and fats also carry important vitamins and nutrients into the bloodstream from the gut. Fat in your food also helps it taste good (a lot of the flavor molecules in food are only soluble in fat) and keeps you sated. And, like protein, fat can slow down the digestion of carbohydrates, so if you eat fat and carbohydrates together, it can prevent some of those sugar highs and lows.

Fat got its bad reputation because it is calorie dense and very easy to digest. It is more than twice as dense in calorie energy as carbohydrates or protein, so it is easy to overdo it. However, some fats are very good for you, and can even help lower your cholesterol levels. These are the unsaturated omega-6 and omega-3 fats found in vegetable oils, olive oil, avocados, nuts, and fish. Omega-3 fats especially have been found to help regulate mood (they have even been used in research as a treatment for major mental illness)[6] and keep your heart healthy.[7] The brain is made up of 60 percent fat, and it is thought that it needs omega-3 fatty acids to work properly. It is easy to see why the omega-3 fats would have some importance in how you think and feel.

Unfortunately, omega-3 fats are very difficult to get in a typical Western diet. The major sources are fish and nuts such as almonds, with flaxseeds being another good source. However, it is not as easy as eating fish every day—most fish is raised in farms, and these fish are not as high in omega-3 as (usually more expensive) wild fish is. Also, a lot of fish have pollutants such as heavy metals, and in order to get enough omega-3 to meet the RDA, you would have to spend a lot of money, and might consume toxic amounts of mercury. (Fish is still a fantastic source of lean protein and omega-3, but the drawbacks of expense and pollution make it difficult to use as your sole source of omega-3 fats.)

Flaxseeds are also problematic. They can be purchased cheaply in bulk at any natural foods grocery store, but they have to be ground (in a coffee grinder, for example) before you can digest them. Also, they contain a form of omega-3 that has to be broken down in the body, and there is some evidence that elderly people especially do not have enough of the right kind of enzyme to break down flax omega-3. You can see why so few Americans eat enough omega-3 fats; but they've been included in some detail here to show how important they are to keep mood steady and the body healthy, and we will return to them in the discussion on supplements, which are the best, most consistent way to get omega-3 fatty acids.

The kinds of fats that have gotten the most media

and medical attention over the years are saturated fats and trans-fats. They are so important to understand that we have created a separate commonsense nutrition rule just for them.

Avoid Saturated Fats and Trans-Fats

It is common knowledge that saturated fats (mostly fats from animal sources, such as beef, bacon, chicken, and dairy) can raise your cholesterol, harden and clog up your arteries, and lead to strokes and heart disease. In fact, the government came out with guidelines that you should eat no more than 10 percent of your total daily calories from saturated fats. If you consider how calorie dense fat is, and how widely available saturated fats are in the American diet (think hamburgers, BBQ pork ribs, cheese, chocolate cake with gooey frosting, ice cream, whole milk...), keeping to this guideline can be a bit of a trick. However, we'll give you some helpful advice about this when we tie all the commonsense nutrition rules together.

The more recent nutrition news has been about the evils of "trans-fats."[8] What are trans-fats? Well, a (very) little biochemistry can help you understand trans-fats and why they are bad for you. Saturated fats from animal sources are congealed at room temperature—think of the fat on beef, or a stick of butter. This gives them some advantages over unsaturated fats (vegetable oils) in creating processed foods of good texture for consumption. The only difference between saturated fats and unsaturated fats is that the former contain some extra hydrogen molecules; saturated fats have hydrogen in enough places to make them "stiffer," so they congeal at a lower temperature. Unsaturated fats like vegetable oils have some spots missing hydrogen, and are therefore floppier and liquid and are sold in bottles as compared to sticks.

The food industry likes the way stiff saturated fats work in making processed foods, but saturated animal fats can be more expensive and messier to get than the fat from vegetables such as soybeans or corn. So food scientists took unsaturated vegetable oils and added hydrogen to make them stiffer—and, voila, trans-fats were born. Anything with "partially hydrogenated" this or that oil is a trans-fat, and you'll find "partially hydrogenated" this or that oil on the ingredients list for most baked snack foods such as chips, cookies, or cupcakes. Trans-fats are also used in the fast food industry for baking and frying.

Why are trans-fats bad? Well, it turns out they are even worse than saturated fats in causing clogged arteries, heart disease, and strokes. Something about the process of adding hydrogen to the natural unsaturated fats causes an unnatural bend in the fat molecules (this unnatural bend is the "trans" part of the trans-fats and this bend seems to be bad for the heart). Trans-fats are everywhere, but should be avoided as much as possible to keep your heart and arteries as healthy as possible. Fortunately, a lot of major food companies have started to phase out trans-fats from their foods, and some of the major fast food giants have said they will stop using them. The government has also stepped in, requiring all food labels to list the amount of trans-fat a food has as of 2006.

Choose the Right Supplements

People who are concerned with health and spend a lot of time looking for heath cures on the Internet can often be the victims of unscrupulous supplement companies.

While some supplements and holistic medicines have been shown to be helpful in certain diseases, the supplement industry is almost completely unregulated. When *Consumer Reports* checked the ingredients of several major supplement brands in May 2004, big differences were often found between the amount of active ingredient on the label and what was actually in the bottle. Some supplements are even dangerous and can interfere with the metabolism of prescription medicines. Prescription and over-the-counter (but pharmaceutical-grade) medicines can also be dangerous, of course, but at least the ingredients are regulated, and pharmacists and doctors can help you in understanding the side effects and risks of taking the medications.

That said, there are some supplements that are important, especially for people with chronic pain and symptoms. Recently, the American government released several new guidelines about vitamins and minerals.[9] Taking an ordinary multivitamin is probably a good idea for everyone (talk to your doctor before taking a vitamin with iron), especially with the average American diet of processed foods stripped of vitamins and minerals. Women of childbearing age should make sure their vitamin has 400 micrograms of folic acid to help prevent neural tube defects in infants. People older than fifty and any vegetarians should make sure their multivitamin contains vitamin B-12. If you don't get any exposure to the sun, you should also make sure the milk you drink or your multivitamin contains vitamin D. Some people with chronic nausea who can't eat well may not get enough vitamins and minerals in what they can eat without extra supplementation. And those who are watching their calories, even while eating healthy foods, can sometimes find it hard to get enough vitamins in their diet.

An omega-3 supplement is also a good idea—the

fish oils used for most supplement capsules are purified and are not contaminated with heavy metals. Bottles of flax oil and capsules are also available as a supplement. In September 2002, the Institute of Medicine of the National Academy of Sciences released a report recommending 1.6 grams per day for men and 1.1 grams per day for women of omega-3 fatty acids.

Finally, those with chronic pain or other symptoms that interfere with the ability to exercise or get around are at special risk for osteoporosis of the bones. For those people and for most women, calcium supplements are important. Calcium carbonate tablets are usually cheapest, but should be taken with food. However, it is difficult for the body to absorb more than about 500 mg at a time, so you should take your tablet with meals that do not contain any dairy products. Also, men should be careful to not have their intake go above 2,500 mg a day, because too much calcium in men can affect prostate health.

How do you know which supplements to buy? There are so many on the market, and supplement companies are not presently regulated to ensure that labels are accurate. However, you can look for brands that carry the U.S. Pharmacopoeia (USP) or National Formulary (NF) notation. These notations mean that the manufacturer has voluntarily complied with a strict set of standards regarding product purity, strength, packaging, and labeling.[10]

After seeing Roy looking so well and fit at the party, Pete decided to make it his New Year's resolution to live healthier. Roy had explained the basic principles he used for eating well and gave Pete a list of books and Internet resources so he could read more. At first it seemed impossible—Pete barely knew how to cook. But Roy's ingredient list was pretty basic: eggs, skinless chicken breasts, cottage cheese, oatmeal, pasta, brown rice, fruits and vegetables, and a few spices.

The first morning of the New Year, Pete cooked an omelet before he went to work. He packed some nuts for snacks to replace the vending machine food, and he brought some tea bags for drinks instead of the two or three cans of soda he consumed during the day. He still went to the fast food restaurant for lunch, but chose the regular-size hamburger instead of the double cheeseburger. That night, his wife stopped by the store and picked up a salad-in-a-bag, and in less than ten minutes, he grilled some chicken breasts for the whole family. At the end of the day, Pete did not feel hungry, or dissatisfied. He slept well, and his stomach pain was no worse and no better.

Putting It All Together

We've just been through the details of all five commonsense nutrition rules. More of the latest reliable information and research on fat, carbohydrates, protein, vitamins, omega-3, and other supplements can be found at the enormous but quite readable National Institutes of Health Office of Dietary Supplements Web site (www.ods.od.nih.gov). Reading about nutrition can get overwhelming, but following the five commonsense rules is meant to be easy. The rules are complementary, so following one will help you in following the next. The most important thing to remember is that what you eat most of the time is important, not what you eat every now and again. The occasional fast food meal, chips, or piece of birthday cake is not something to feel guilty about. And remember, just following one or two of the rules at a time can have positive effects on your nutrition and energy levels. Good nutrition is not an all-or-nothing endeavor.

Just as we are bombarded with health information in our society, we are also constantly seeing advertisements for highly refined, less healthy foods. They are everywhere—at the end of every grocery aisle and in vending machines at every major public gathering place. And just as we have learned how to filter out the excess and hyped-up health information, it is important to slowly learn to go back to the commonsense basics when it comes to eating, most of the time.

Here are the rules again:

1. Eat small amounts frequently throughout the day, starting with breakfast.

2. Eat unprocessed, natural foods as much as possible.

3. Eat a variety of nutrients in a variety of colors.

4. Avoid saturated fats and trans-fats.

5. Choose the right supplements.

First of all, to follow all these rules at once and completely change the way you eat can seem overwhelming. Usually, the easiest one to start with is eating frequently in small sizes. For example, if you get a submarine sandwich and a package of chips at lunchtime, eat half of your meal at lunch and save half of it for around three p.m. That way you avoid stuffing yourself at lunchtime (causing the midafternoon energy slump and drowsiness), and you get a pick-me-up meal to last you until dinnertime. This afternoon snack can help keep you from being ravenous before dinner and help prevent predinner binges on calorie-dense foods like chips and ice cream.

Once you've tried eating more frequently, you can start to substitute in natural foods. Instead of a candy bar at ten a.m., try an apple or two. Use whole-grain bread for your sandwiches instead of white bread. For a sweet treat, try low-fat yogurt or no-sugar-added fudge popsicles instead of ice cream or pastries. You'll notice that by eating more natural foods, you will automatically avoid trans-fats and also many saturated fats.

Getting a variety of foods in a variety of colors can be difficult. It often takes some planning to follow this rule, doing your own cooking or spending some time studying the best combinations of the most natural foods at your favorite restaurants or convenience stores. If you feel ready to jump in, the easiest way to follow most of the rules at once is to plan meals based on variety and portion size, and take it from there. Most of your meals should have a lean protein, a complex carbohydrate, and/or a fruit or vegetable. Each portion size should be anywhere from 250–400 calories for women (a lower amount for smaller, less active women and six meals a day) and 350–500 calories for men. Obviously these are averages—if you are underweight or extremely muscular or active, you may need more food. The lower limit of a healthy number of calories per day for an inactive adult is around 1,200; below that, it is extremely difficult to get the nutrients you need to stay energized and avoid nutritional deficiencies.

A typical meal of 250–500 calories is about half a cup or 3–4 ounces of lean protein (half a can of tuna, for example), a cup of complex carbohydrate (a small baked potato), and, for most meals, one fruit or unlimited vegetables. You'll notice that potatoes and corn, traditionally thought of as vegetables, have a lot more in common nutritionally with grains than with fibrous vegetables like broccoli. Therefore, corn and potatoes are in the complex-carb category. Remember, you get five to six of these meals a day for optimal energy and to avoid any metabolic slowdowns. If you like to have a bigger dinner, make the snacks 50–100 calories.

Here is a table to make following the food rules easier. (The list of foods is by no means exhaustive—you'll find the lean protein is the most limited category; there are unbelievable varieties of starches, fruits, and vegetables available at most grocery stores.)

Protein	Complex Carb	Fruits and Veggies	Sweets/Fats
Use about half a cup in most meals—an average serving would be 3 ounces for a woman and 4 ounces for a man.	This serving size is about a cup per meal.	Eat as many vegetables as you want, and up to 3–4 fruits per day.	Use in small amounts.
Lean beef cuts Lean ground beef Skinless chicken breast Lean ground turkey Turkey breast Low-fat cottage cheese Soy burger patty Textured soy Fish and seafood Egg whites String cheese* Buffalo, ostrich Nuts such as almonds—eat up to ¼ cup a day *not lean, but inexpensive, and easy to carry around for a quick snack. One stick is about 80 calories.	Potatoes Yams Corn Beans Rice Brown rice Oatmeal Skim milk Fat-free yogurt Pasta Bread Quinoa Bulgur wheat	Squash Peas Apples Oranges Pears Broccoli Asparagus Cucumber Cabbage Lettuce Peppers Green beans Blueberries Salsa Tomato Bananas	Honey Oils Egg yolks Light maple syrup **Supplements** Multivitamin Omega-3 Calcium

For example, for breakfast you might take your multivitamin, omega-3, and calcium supplement. Have ½ cup oatmeal microwaved with ¼ cup fresh blueberries and ¾ cup water and a teaspoon of maple syrup. Add an egg-white omelet (four whites, one yolk) made in a nonstick pan, and you have a hearty, healthy breakfast that is about 300 calories and only 6 percent saturated fat. By choosing lean cuts of meat, soy products, and low-fat or fat-free dairy, you can avoid saturated fats and trans-fats. By choosing something from each of the major categories, you eat a variety of nutrients in a variety of colors. And by eating frequently and controlling your portion sizes, you will be fully energized throughout the day without being too full or feeling hungry.

A midmorning snack might be an apple and string cheese, and lunch could be a turkey breast sandwich on whole-wheat bread with mustard, lettuce, and tomato. At three in the afternoon, have a container of fat-free yogurt. Dinner can be chicken breast, squash, and brown rice. If you eat a little more during one meal, make up for it with smaller portions the next meal. Nuts can be filling on their own as a midmorning or midafternoon snack, but if you are trying to lose weight, it is important not to eat more than $\frac{1}{4}$ cup at a time (about fifteen almonds), or the calories can add up quickly.

An easy and inexpensive way to eat according to the commonsense nutrition rules is to cook up four to eight servings at a time of several meals, store the extra as premade meal servings in the refrigerator or freezer, and eat the leftovers for the next few days. Most health and fitness magazines will have tasty recipes that adhere to the commonsense nutrition rules. Even standards such as macaroni and cheese can be made to fit this model—cook it as directed, add a can of tuna and a bag of frozen vegetables until everything is heated through, and use the box to make eight servings instead of four.

If there is a party on Friday night or a neighborhood BBQ on Saturday, by all means enjoy yourself and have the yummy food available there. It is what you eat most of the time that matters, not the occasional bowl of ice cream.

And, finally, if you don't feel like making drastic changes to your diet right now, don't. These guidelines are meant to help, not to make you feel guilty. It is *not* a diet that you must follow to the letter or feel like a failure. The main goal of these commonsense nutrition rules is to give you some information about how to eat for consistent energy levels, to feel healthy, to get enough vitamins and good fats, and to try to sort out some of the confusing hype about carbohydrates, proteins, and fats.

After four or five weeks of eating well, Pete realized it had been several days since he felt his stomach pains. He went to the doctor again, and the scale reported a loss of ten pounds. His doctor approved him going off his stomach medicine, and he found that even without the medicine, his pain was nearly gone. Roy had told Pete that ever since he started eating mostly natural, healthy foods, he stopped getting the bronchitis he used to have every winter. Pete noticed that when his kids came home with colds from school, he seemed less likely to get them. He attributed this stronger resistance to his new way of eating.

Exercise: What to Do and How to Begin

Just as the right nutrition can improve your health and energy levels, so can the right exercise. It boosts your metabolism, helps you maintain a healthy weight, reduces stress, helps your heart stay in shape, and helps you stay strong enough to do your daily activities as easily as possible. And just as food comes in three varieties (carbohydrates, protein, and fats), a complete exercise program has three basic components: cardiovascular exercise, weight training, and flexibility training.

As with any topic related to health these days, there are countless dissenting opinions on the best kind of exercise, when it should be done, where, how much…an Internet search of "weight training" yields more than five million results! Our purpose is to give you a starting point and to explain some of the benefits of each part of a complete exercise program.

Roy didn't improve his asthma and lose sixty pounds by changing his diet alone; he also relied on exercise. He told Pete which gym he joined, and Pete, with the doctor's enthusiastic approval, made an appointment with one of the staff members, who designed an initial program for him. Pete was pretty skeptical—a couple of times he'd tried taking up running, but after the first few days of side stitches, gasping breath, and aching shins, he'd decided he was better off getting that extra hour of sleep in the morning.

At the gym, just like at the doctor's office, Pete got his weight and blood pressure checked. The friendly staff member made some recommendations about how to begin, and showed him how to use several exercise machines in the cardiovascular and weight areas of the gym. He told Pete to start slowly—consistency was more important than pushing his limits at first.

Cardiovascular Exercise

Before you start on any exercise program, it is imperative that your symptoms first be evaluated by a doctor. Once it is determined that your persistent symptoms are benign, or part of a disorder that can benefit from exercise, it is safe to begin (with your doctor's direction). For almost everyone, increasing physical activity is a step in the right direction for improving health. The more inactive you are, the more a moderate increase in your activity will help lower your mortality.[11]

Walking, running, bicycling, elliptical training—any physical activity that raises your heart rate and keeps it there for a while is considered cardiovascular exercise. This is the kind of exercise that strengthens your heart and lungs,[12] burns calories, and decreases bad cholesterol.[13] If done long enough with a high enough intensity, it can cause the release of natural endorphins, which ease pain and anxiety. By increasing your stamina through cardiovascular exercise, the less vigorous activities of your life such as shopping and climbing stairs become easier.

The American Heart Association recommends that children, adolescents, and adults participate in at least sixty minutes of activity every day. Older adults and people with disabilities can also get significant benefits from being active as much as possible. The activities don't have to be strenuous—walking, using a nonmotorized wheelchair, gardening, golfing, and climbing stairs instead of taking the elevator all work. Each little bit of extra activity will help to increase your stamina and well-being. Sixty minutes may sound like a lot, but the guidelines are meant to count *all* your activity throughout the day. That means parking your car at the far end of the parking lot and giving yourself five more minutes of walking to the store each way counts as part of your sixty minutes. Taking the stairs instead of the escalator or elevator gives you more minutes, too. Even fidgeting in your chair at work or standing up in between meetings can help you from putting on extra pounds in the long run.

If you decide to start regular cardiovascular exercise, the first step is to figure out what to do, and how much of it you should do. There is no single number or intensity that is right for everyone; each person has his or her own level of fitness at any particular moment. For one person, walking halfway down the block may be difficult, for another it might be running an eight-minute mile. Walking is a terrific starting point—it is inexpensive, easy, and low risk. A good level of exertion is a brisk enough walk so that you can still talk, but it would be difficult to sing. By adding distance and intensity (via hills, for example), you can slowly build up your stamina and improve your health.

Common sense is just as important for cardiovascular exercise as it is for nutrition. Check with your doctor about the exercises that are safe for your medical conditions, keep yourself hydrated, wear appropriate clothing, and don't go out into extremely hot or cold weather if you are not used to it. And don't start with five miles if you haven't been active for a while. Also, change up your workout every once in a while to be sure you don't get too used to one particular activity or overuse one set of muscles.

Weight Training

The basic health benefits and practice of cardiovascular exercise have been heavily publicized and presented in the past two decades. More recently, however, the benefits of a program of weight training have also been touted, especially for the elderly and the disabled.

Weight training, also known as strength or resistance training, may bring to mind pictures of bodybuilders and enormous barbells, but in fact many kinds of exercise, such as circuit training, pilates, and yoga, have elements of weight training in them. In general, participating in a regular program of weight training can help adults improve overall health and fitness, increase muscular strength, and improve bone density. For older adults, weight training is recommended to decrease the risk of falls and fractures, and to promote independent living.[14]

For those of you with chronic pain that restricts the amount of moving around you do, weight training can be an important tool to keep your bones strong. Older or inactive adults can improve strength by orders of magnitude in a relatively short amount of time. Research has shown that pain from osteoarthritis of the knee can decreased by as much as 43 percent with resistance training.[15] For those with diabetes, a recent study showed dramatic improvements in glucose control with sixteen weeks of weight training.[16] Strength training has also been shown to improve mood, help insomnia, and increase cardiac health.[17]

Why does weight training have so many benefits? There are two reasons: it makes you strong, and it makes you lean. Building muscles means adding lean mass, and the more muscle you have, the more calories you burn doing just about anything. This keeps the amount of fat you have under better control.

If you are a woman and are afraid of "bulking up," don't be. Very few women have the genetic makeup to become like the large-muscled female bodybuilders you might have seen on television or in magazines. Women simply don't have enough testosterone (without taking anabolic steroids, which are obviously not recommended) to gain huge amounts of muscle from strength training. It will, however, make you leaner, and when combined with proper exercise and nutrition is the key to getting to and maintaining a healthy weight.

Beginning a weight training program is easy—as long as you have an appropriate guide. If you belong to a gym, ask someone who works there to design an initial program for you and show you all the exercises with the correct form. Exercise videos should have good cues to keep you from injuring yourself, work your muscles in a balanced way, and give reasonable ways for you to know how hard to work and how much to lift. Any general bookstore will have many different books about weight training, many of which are complete with diagrams and explanations. The end of this chapter also lists several reliable resources available for free on the Internet.

Just as with nutrition and cardiovascular exercise, variety in resistance training is important to keep the workout challenging and interesting, and decrease the chance of overuse injuries.

Flexibility Training

Flexibility training is often overlooked as a component of a complete exercise program. Fortunately, it is the easiest piece to begin and can be done by everyone, even those with chronic pain that limits other activities. Stretching prevents injury, increases range of motion, improves posture, and reduces stress. It is the perfect adjunct to the relaxation training we described in previous chapters.

There are a few safety principles you need to know before beginning a regular program of stretching:

1. Use static stretching; don't bounce.

2. Never stretch a cold muscle; always warm up first.

3. Stretch during and after cardiovascular and weight training sessions.

A static stretch means you slowly elongate your muscles through the full range of motion and hold for fifteen to thirty seconds in the furthest comfortable position. Stop if you experience pain. Don't hold your breath; just keep inhaling and exhaling naturally as the muscles lengthen. Stretching all the major muscle groups in this fashion helps the soreness and knots caused by regular exercise and activities.

Trying to stretch a cold muscle is difficult and can even cause injury. If stretching is the only exercise you do, do it in the afternoon or at the end of the day. Otherwise, do five to ten minutes of warmup (whatever activity you will be doing, such as walking or cycling), stretch, and then continue at a more intense workout pace. Stretching in this way ensures that your muscles are flexible and helps to prevent injury.

Flexibility training after the workout will prevent some soreness, and stretching the muscles while they are at their warmest will give you the largest range of motion and the best stretch. The postworkout stretch is one way to feel fantastic without any side effects or expense.

The President's Council on Physical Fitness and Sports recommends stretching daily if possible, but at least three times a week, for approximately ten to twelve minutes.[18] It goes further to recommend four to five stretches for each major muscle group, each held for fifteen to thirty seconds.

Correct form is important for proper stretching in order to prevent injury. Consult fitness magazines, books, or demonstrations from fitness professionals to make sure you get a complete stretching program that places balanced emphasis on all major muscles and avoids any stretches that might cause injury (such as the "hurdle stretch" used years ago).

Pete began a slow but steady program of exercise. After getting home from work and just before dinner, he walked several miles. A couple days a week he made time to go to the gym and lift weights. Sometimes he went with Roy, and they lifted together. He made sure he stretched during and after every workout. He enjoyed new stamina, and switched from walking to jogging, and then tried jumping rope. Finally, he quit smoking. He wanted to be able to run faster and farther, and felt his smoking kept him from doing his best.

By his thirty-sixth birthday, Pete had lost twenty pounds. He could run three miles without stopping in less than half an hour. His blood pressure dropped, and his doctor approved him going off his medication. His stomach never bothered him anymore.

Sometimes Pete skipped a workout, or ate a big pile of chips, or drank a few too many beers watching football. But the next day he would continue on with his plan of healthy eating and exercise. He had never felt better in his life.

For more information from a reliable source on cardiovascular exercise, weight training, stretches, and even how to order a free exercise guide, you can try the National Institutes of Health at www.nia.nih.gov/exercisebook. Another good resource with strength training programs and plenty of free health information is from Tufts University, at www.strongwomen.com and the National Center for Chronic Disease Prevention and Health Promotion, Division of Nutrition and Physical Activity, at www.cdc .gov/nccdphp/dnpa. Cross-referenced videos of nearly every weight training exercise can be found at www.exrx .net/exercise.html.

CHAPTER TEN

Four Final Principles

You cannot simply turn off a symptom or a bodily sensation any more than you can ignore the annoying cell phone conversation of the man standing beside you in an elevator. But you can alter your reactions to your symptoms, change your thoughts about them, demystify them, and make them less frightening. Doing this diminishes the discomfort surrounding the symptom and gives you a crucial sense of control over it. Although you can't determine whether or not you become ill or develop symptoms, you can control how much they bother you and how much they disrupt your life. You can learn to manage them better. This is what coping is all about. By understanding how social pressures around you shape your expectations and your feelings, doing the exercises in the preceding chapters, and learning ways of healthy living, you have developed and practiced a personalized coping system for your specific symptoms.

In our work helping patients to overcome symptoms that persist even after their doctors have done their best to diagnose and treat them, we have discovered four underlying principles that are helpful in developing a deeper understanding of the meaning of symptoms. In this concluding chapter, we discuss each of these principles.

"Curable Pain Is Unbearable Pain"[1]

The esteemed psychiatrist Elvin Semrad observed, "The things people suffer most from are the things they tell themselves that are not true." (In a similar vein he also remarked, "Pretending that it can be when it can't is how people break their hearts.") Many of us cling to the idea that our symptoms could be cured if only we could find just the right specialist, gain access to the latest experimental drug, or undergo some miraculous new surgical procedure. Do you keep searching for an outright cure for your symptoms? Do you believe the cure exists, but that you simply haven't found it yet? Do you spend your energy scrutinizing your body for additional clues to the ever-elusive diagnosis, spend your money on unfounded medical cures, and spend your time waiting and wishing your problem would go away entirely?

This is a trap that intensifies symptoms. Pain that we believe can be assuaged, that we think is unnecessary, and that we feel we shouldn't have to bear hurts more than pain we know is unavoidable. "Curable pain is unbearable pain," as Ivan Illich has pointed out.[2] Pain and discomfort are most excruciating just when the relief we have been expecting has failed to materialize. The pain of your fractured ankle becomes agonizing after you've swallowed a pain pill but it hasn't taken effect yet.

Something similar happens with chronic illness: if you believe your infirmity is treatable and that the symptoms are therefore avoidable and unnecessary, they seem more burdensome and more severe. Curable pain seems to be unbearable pain. Once you believe your arthritic hands shouldn't hurt as much as they do—that relief would be forthcoming if only you got the latest breakthrough treatment or found just the right specialist—then the aching and stiffness become intolerable. Unfounded optimism makes it harder to live with the ailments that in fact are not curable. As strange as it sounds, the first step in overcoming refractory symptoms is to acknowledge that they are indeed refractory and aren't simply going to disappear. The first step to take in beginning to feel better is to come to an acceptance of your illness and to give up on illusory, phantom cures.

The Paradox of Surrender

There is a great paradox inherent in overcoming our symptoms: in order to cope successfully with them, we must first acknowledge that we are stuck with them. To put it simply, you don't learn to cope with adversity until you acknowledge that you will have to. The paradox is that the very acceptance of this plight opens the door to improving it. Many gravely ill people feel better and are less impaired than healthy hypochondriacs. Why? Because they have accepted the reality of their situation, and have therefore set about making the best of it. They know nothing more is to be gained by seeking an illusory cure, and so they turn their efforts to coping with their illness, managing it, compensating for it, and overcoming it.

Only when we accept the harsh reality that we are just going to have to live with an illness can we begin to make the best of it. This is the paradox of surrender. As long as we expect to be cured of a malady, we are detained from the business of learning to minimize it, deal with it, and cope with it—after all, why should we, since it will soon go away? And the coping process is what ultimately makes discomfort tolerable. This is as true of the hypochondriac as it is of someone with chronic fatigue or allergies or psoriasis or cancer. Thus patients find their afflictions, both serious and trivial, less excruciating once they frankly acknowledge them and then set about learning to live with them.

When we come to terms with the reality of our ailments and accept the fact that we are stuck with them, something quite surprising often happens: the symptoms turn out to be more tolerable and less fearsome than we had imagined. The reality, as we've seen in Chapter 9, is that many people find they are able to cope very successfully with very serious illnesses and impairments, once they put their minds to it. But we don't put our minds to coping with our ailments until we acknowledge that we are just going to have to. We don't develop the skills to overcome something until we admit that there is something we have to overcome. In short, you can't *feel better* until you accept the fact that you won't *get better.*

Once people accept the reality of the obstacles they face, they can often deal with them remarkably well, even heroically, and with greater success than they ever thought themselves capable of. Gladys Rogers is a sixty-six-year-old widowed grandmother. Trained as a librarian, she stopped working to raise her two daughters, and then returned to work part time when they were older. Her husband died six years ago, and soon after, she developed breast cancer. She and her doctors were optimistic about her prognosis following a mastectomy, but after only a year her cancer returned. Though chemotherapy slowed the progression of her disease, it did not halt it.

The last year has been a frightening, depressing, and painful one, but Gladys has come to accept the fact that her future is limited. And since then, she has found meaning and significance in her life, along with a sense of peace. She has used her illness and the knowledge that her life is finite to help her focus on and live in the present. Although she continues to have serious symptoms, particularly weakness, fatigue, and back pain, they

do not dominate her life. She maintains a hopeful attitude by setting realistic and proximate goals, such as seeing the flowering bulbs she planted last fall bloom again
this spring, and seeing her granddaughter play the lead
role in her grade school drama production. Gladys has
become more observant and appreciative of the simple,
daily events around her—things she used to take for
granted—like going to the movies with a friend and
hearing the beauty of the church choir each Sunday. She
has discovered pleasure and satisfaction in the small details of everyday life. It is not the peak experiences like
winning the lottery that make us happy over the long
run, but a good joke at the dinner table with your family,
the beautiful fall foliage on a tree in the backyard, a
good serve in tennis, or petting your dog.

Gladys has found that her illness and her approach-
ing death make her more compassionate toward others,
more forgiving of their foibles, and less irritable. Though
she used to get very irritated with her grandson's lack of
"manners," especially the way he wore his baseball cap
indoors, it now no longer bothers her. She says, "It's just
not important enough to get mad about."

Gladys is making a videotape for her family in which
she tells them all about her life and her childhood. It is a
kind of gift she is giving them, a way to tell them about
their family's history and a way for them to appreciate
and remember her. She has even consented to be inter-
viewed by her oncologist as part of a class he teaches to
help medical students better understand what it is like to
live with a terminal illness.

So it is possible to cope remarkably well, even with
the most serious disorders and the most distressing symptoms. And coping begins by acknowledging what you are
up against; only then can you begin to make the best of it.

No One Gets Out of Here Alive

It is also helpful to see symptoms and illness in a broader context. When we get sick, it often seems to us as if we have been victimized, unfairly singled out and personally targeted for misfortune. This sense of injustice, unfairness, and victimization only makes matters worse. But the reality is that none of us is exempted from illness and disease, because they are an endemic part of the human predicament. Illness is an inextricable element of life and not something for which you have been singled out; it is not evidence of uniquely bad luck or of mistreatment at the hands of fate, or of an injustice visited upon you alone. You're not different from everyone else in this respect. We all get sick, and we all die. Remember, "No one gets out of here alive." (Or, as another wag has put it, the death rate is one per person.)

It is profoundly reassuring to realize that you are not alone in this sense. The value of this lesson is attested to by the power of patient support groups. Participants find these groups enormously comforting precisely because they learn that they are not alone, that others face similar impairments, setbacks, and obstacles.

It is important to share with and get to know others who face difficulties like yours, because they can be a reference point that helps you put your own situation in perspective. And as we've seen in Chapter 2, how ill you feel is powerfully shaped by whom you compare yourself to. When you compare yourself to an ideal of vigor and youth and perfect health, you are bound to feel worse; but when you compare yourself to others who suffer and struggle as you do, you feel less alone and less unfortunate.

Consider two patients seen during a typical morning's busy medical practice. They compare themselves to very different standards of good health and therefore feel very differently about their illnesses. The first, Barbara Edwards, is a fifty-four-year-old grandmother with progressive, severe rheutmatoid arthritis. She comes in for a scheduled visit and does not volunteer any complaints. When asked how she is doing overall, she notes that every time she visits her doctor she sees other patients who appear to be "worse off" than she, and this makes her feel that her problems really aren't that bad after all. When closely questioned, however, she confesses that her hands are stiff, her feet ache when she walks, and she feels tired a lot of the time. She even admits that her symptoms are "pretty bad some days," but adds quickly that her medications help somewhat and that she remains upbeat; Barbara is particularly looking forward to a visit from her grandchildren next month. She is tranquil, friendly, likes her doctor, and is grateful for his help.

The doctor's next patient is Ethel Blackwood, also a fifty-four-year-old grandmother of two, who is also bothered by fatigue, joint pain, and aching muscles. Yet in Ethel's case, an extensive diagnostic evaluation has not disclosed any serious medical disease—she is basically a healthy woman. She ruminates about younger family members with seemingly boundless energy and thinks about the robust and glamorous models she sees in advertisements for vitamins and hair coloring. Compared to them, it seems to her that she is very ill and doing poorly. Ethel's symptoms distress her and interfere with almost every aspect of her life; she feels so sick that she avoids her friends because she is "no fun to be with." She feels that her affliction is very unfair, and she is dissatisfied with her doctor because he has not been able to relieve her symptoms.

Two fifty-four-year-old grandmothers with the same symptoms and the same doctor; one is sick but feels well, the other well but feels sick. They make it clear that it is possible to cope remarkably well with very serious disease and, conversely, to be crippled by symptoms that aren't medically serious at all. How ill you feel is profoundly influenced by the people you choose to compare yourself to. Barbara is grateful that she is better off than many of the patients she sees sitting in the waiting room. Ethel is angry and resentful because her health seems so much worse than the models in advertisements. Comparing yourself to those who are sick can make your current state seem more tolerable, and comparing yourself to an ideal of good health and youth and vigor can leave you feeling worse.

This is an important point, because feeling that your illness is an injustice for which you have been singled out and uniquely afflicted makes the illness seem worse. Now you not only experience bodily distress, but you also feel mistreated and outraged. Your illness is an insult, a source of indignation because it seems like an undeserved misfortune. If you think that you should not have gotten sick, and believe that someone or something is at fault and responsible for it, it makes your symptoms worse. So it is helpful to see your situation and your health in a realistic context, to compare yourself to real people with their own fair share of setbacks and struggles and misfortunes. Remember: No one gets out of here alive.

Health Is a Means to an End

Finally, people cope better with illnesses and lessen their symptoms when they realize that good health is a means to an end, not an end in itself. Physical well-being is not an adequate substitute for a gratifying, complete, and rewarding life. The most important thing about good health is that it enables you to pursue a more satisfying and rewarding life—to work productively, to play with your children, pursue your hobbies, participate in the charitable effort going on at your church, travel abroad and see the world.[3] But it is not a *substitute* for these things; it can only enable you to pursue them. "How well people manage lives marked by illness depends not on the nature of the illness but on the strength of their conviction that life is worth living no matter what complications are imposed on it."[4]

Less than perfect health is not in itself a failure or defeat, or someone's fault, but rather an obstacle that interferes with our ability to accomplish the important things in life. Our primary goal should be living successfully, not striving for perfect physical health. If we find more meaning in our work and our relationships, experience a fuller emotional and spiritual life, derive pleasure from play and from our pastimes, then we are better prepared to deal with ill health. We need *reasons* to overcome our symptoms and to ignore them. We must have something important that needs doing. Some people find that sense of purpose and meaning in religious devotion, in professional accomplishment, in raising children, or in the intimacy and companionship of a loving marriage.

We hope that the lesson chapters in this book have helped you to learn to live with your medical symptoms. Our purpose is to help you develop methods to enhance your life in spite of pain, fatigue, anxiety, and insomnia. Through the techniques and exercises in the proceeding chapters, you can stop suffering, gain control over your symptoms, and then be free to live a more satisfying life.

Notes ————————————————————

Chapter 1

1. Barsky, AJ, Ahern, DK. "Cognitive Behavior Therapy for Hypochondriasis: A Randomized Controlled Trial." *JAMA* 2004; 291:1464–70.

Chapter 2

1. Wildavsky, A. "Doing Better and Feeling Worse: The Political Pathology of Health Policy." In Knowles, JH, editor, *Doing Better and Feeling Worse: Health in the United States*. New York: W. W. Norton and Co., 1977: 105–23.

2. Barsky, AJ. "The Paradox of Health." *New Engl J Med* 1988; 318:414–18.

3. Verbrugge, LM, Ascione, FJ. "Exploring the Iceberg: Common Symptoms and How People Care for Them." *Med Care* 1987; 25:539–69. Hannay, DR. *The Symptom Iceberg: A Study of Community Health*. London: Routledge & Kegan Paul, 1979. Barsky, AJ. *Worried Sick: Our Troubled Quest for Wellness*. Boston:

Little, Brown & Co., 1988. Hammond, EC. "Some Preliminary Findings on Physical Complaints from a Prospective Study of 1,064,004 Men and Women." *Am J Pub Health* 1964; 54:11–23.

4. Chen, M. "The Epidemiology of Self-Perceived Fatigue Among Adults." *Prev Med* 1986; 15:74–81. Shefer, A, Dobbins, JG, Fukuda, K, Steele, L, Koo, D, Nisenbaum, R, et al. "Fatiguing Illness Among Employees in Three Large State Office Buildings, California 1993: Was There an Outbreak?" *J Psychiatric Res* 1996; 31:31–43. Pawlikowska, T, Chalder, T, Hirsch, SR, Wallace, P, Wright, DJM, Wessely, SC. "Population Based Study of Fatigue and Psychological Distress." *Br Med J* 1994; 308:763–66. Buchwald, D, Umali, J, Kith, P, Pearlman, T, Komaroff, AL. "Chronic Fatigue and the Chronic Fatigue Syndrome: Prevalence in a Pacific Northwest Health Care System." *Ann Intern Med* 1995; 123:81–88.

5. Loney, P, Stratford, PW. "The Prevalence of Low Back Pain in Adults: A Methodological Review of the Literature." *Physical Therapy* 1999; 79:384–96.

6. Woodwell, DA. *National Ambulatory Care Medical Survey: 1998 Summary*. Hyattsville, MD, National Center for Health Statistics, Centers for Disease Control and Prevention.

7. Gruenberg, MM. "The Failures of Success." *Millbank Mem Fund Quart* 1977; 55:3–24.

8. Keeney, RL. "Decisions about Life-Threatening Risks." *New Engl J Med* 1994; 331:193–96.

9. Barsky, AJ. "The Paradox of Health." Barsky, AJ. *Worried Sick.*

10. Center for Communicable Disease; National Center for Chronic Disease Prevention and Health Promotion: Health Related Quality of Life; Nationwide Trend.

11. Ibid.

12. Barsky, AJ. *Worried Sick.* Palmer, KT, Wash, K, Bendall, H, Cooper, C, Coggon, D. "Back Pain in Britain: Comparison of Two Prevalence Surveys at an Interval of 10 Years." *Br Med J* 2000; 320:1577–78. Wessely, S. "Chronic Fatigue Syndrome: A 20th Century Illness?" *Scand J Work Environ Health* 1997; 23:17–34. Anderson, DW, Morrison, EM. "The Worth of Medical Care." *Med Care Rev* 1989; 46:121–56.

13. Ursin, H. "Sensitization, Somatization, and Subjective Health Complaints." *Int'l J Behav Med* 1997; 4:105–16.

14. Robertson, JT. "The Rape of the Spine." *Surg Neurol* 1993; 39:5–12.

15. Ursin, H. "Sensitization."

16. Bellamy, R. "Compensation Neurosis: Financial Reward for Illness as Nocebo." *Clin Orth Rel Res* 1997; 336:94–106. Robertson, LS, Keeve, JP. "Worker Injuries: The Effects of Workers' Compensation and OSHA Inspections." *Journal of Health Politics, Policy & Law* 1983; 8:581–97.

17. Eisenberg, DM, Davis, RB, Ettner, SL, Appel, S, Wilkey, S, Van Rompay, M, et al. "Trends in Alternative Medicine Use in the United States, 1990–1997: Results of a Follow-Up National Survey." *JAMA* 1998; 280:1569–75. Astin, JA. "Why Patients Use Alternative Medicine: Results of a National Study." *JAMA* 1998; 279:1548–53.

18. Eisenberg, DM, et al., "Trends in Alternative Medicine."

19. Ibid.

20. Price, DD. "Psychological and Neural Mechanisms of the Affective Dimension of Pain." *Science* 2000; 288:1769–72.

21. Rainville, P, Duncan, GH, Price, DD, Carrier, B, Bushnell, MC. "Pain Affect Encoded in Human Anterior Cingulate but not Somatosensory Cortex." *Science* 1997; 277:968–71.

22. Ibid.

23. Loney, P, Stratford, PW. "The Prevalence of Low Back Pain."

24. Jensen, MC, Brant-Zawadzki, MN, Obuchowski, N, Modic, MT, Malkasian, D, Ross, JS. "Magnetic Resonance Imaging of the Lumbar Spine in People Without Back Pain." *New Engl J Med* 1994; 331:69–73.

25. Barsky, AJ, Cleary, PD, Barnett, MC, Christiansen, CL, Ruskin, JN. "The Accuracy of Symptom Reporting in Patients Complaining of Palpitations." *Am*

J Med 1994; 97:214–21. Barsky, AJ. "Palpitations, Arrhythmias, and Awareness of Cardiac Activity." *Ann Intern Med* 2001; 134:832–37.

26. Kroenke, K, Spitzer, RL, deGruy, FV, Hahn, SR, Linzer, M, Williams, JBW, et al. "Multisomatoform Disorder: An Alternative to Undifferentiated Somatoform Disorder for the Somatizing Patient in Primary Care." *Arch Gen Psychiat* 1997; 54:352–58. Kroenke, K. "Studying Symptoms: Sampling and Measurement Issues." *Ann Intern Med* 2001; 134: 844–53.

27. Kroenke, K, Mangelsdorff, AD. "Common Symptoms in Ambulatory Care: Incidence, Evaluation, Therapy, and Outcome." *Am J Med* 1989; 86:262–66. Kroenke, K, Spitzer, RL, Williams, JBW, Linzer, M, Hahn, SR, deGruy, FV, et al. "Physical Symptoms in Primary Care: Predictors of Psychiatric Disorders and Functional Impairment." *Arch Fam Med* 1994; 3:774–79. Martina, B, Bucheli, B, Stotz, M, Battegay, E, Gyr, N. "First Clinical Judgment by Primary Care Physicians Distinguishes Well Between Nonorganic and Organic Causes of Abdominal or Chest Pain." *J Gen Int Med* 1997; 12:459–65.

28. Potts, SG, Bass, CM. "Psychosocial Outcome and Use of Medical Resources in Patients with Chest Pain and Normal or Near-Normal Coronary Arteries: A Long-Term Follow-Up Study." *Quart J Med* 1993; 86: 583–93. Isner, JM, Salem, DN, Banas, JS, Levine, HJ. "Long-Term Clinical Course of Patients with Normal Coronary Arteriography: Follow-Up Study of 121 Patients with Normal or Nearly Normal Coronary Arteriograms." *Am Heart J* 1981; 102: 645–53.

29.   Lichtenberg, PA, Skehan, MW, Swensen, CH. "The
      Role of Personality, Recent Life Stress and Arthritic
      Severity in Predicting Pain." *J Psychosom Res* 1984;
      28:231–36. Lichtenberg, PA, Swensen, CH, Skehan,
      MW. "Further Investigations of the Role of Personal-
      ity Lifestyle and Arthritic Severity in Predicting Pain."
      J Psychosom Res 1986; 30:327–37.

30.   Alonso, J, Anto, JM, Gonzalez, M, Fiz, JA, Izqui-
      erdo, J, Morera, J. "Measurement of General Health
      Status of Non-Oxygen-Dependent Chronic Ob-
      structive Pulmonary Disease Patients." *Med Care*
      1992; 30:MS125–MS135. Burdon, JGW, Juniper, EF,
      Killian, KJ, Hargreave, FE, Campbell, EJM. "The
      Perception of Breathlessness in Asthma." *Am Rev
      Respir Dis* 1982; 126:825–28. Mahler, DA, Matthay,
      RA, Snyder, PE, Wells, CK, Loke, J. "Sustained-
      Release Theophylline Reduces Dyspnea in Nonre-
      versible Obstructive Airway Disease." *Am Rev Respir
      Dis* 1985; 131:22–25. Mahler, DA, Weinberg, DH,
      Wells, CK, Feinstein, AR. "The Measurement of
      Dyspnea: Contents Interobserver Agreement, and
      Physiologic Correlates of Two New Clinical In-
      dexes." *Chest* 1984; 85:751–58.

31.   Frimodt-Moller, PC, Jensen, KM, Iversen, P, Madsen,
      PO, Bruskewitz, RC. "Analysis of Presenting Symp-
      toms in Prostatism." *J Urol* 1984; 132:272–76.

32.   Dwosh, IL, Giles, AR, Ford, PM, Pater, JL, Anas-
      tassiades, TP. "Plasmapheresis Therapy in Rheuma-
      toid Arthritis." *New Engl J Med* 1983; 308:1124–29.

33.   Peterson, WL, Sturdevant, RA, Frankl, HD, Rich-
      ardson, CT, Isenberg, JI, Elashoff, JD, et al. "Healing

of Duodenal Ulcer with an Antacid Regimen." *New Engl J Med* 1977; 297:341–45.

34. Wood, MM, Elwood, PC. "Symptoms of Iron Deficiency Anaemia: A Community Survey." *Br J Prev Soc Med* 1966; 20:117–21.

35. Barsky, AJ. "Amplification, Somatization and the Somatoform Disorders." *Psychosomatics* 1992; 33:28–34. Barsky, AJ, Goodson, JD, Lane, RS, Cleary, PD. "The Amplification of Somatic Symptoms." *Psychosom Med* 1988; 50:510–19.

36. Ibid.

37. Brickman, P, Coates, D, Janoff-Bulman, R. "Lottery Winners and Accident Victims: Is Happiness Relative?" *J Personal Soc Psychol* 1978; 36:917–27.

38. Breetvelt, IS, van Dam, FSAM. "Underreporting by Cancer Patients: The Case of Response-Shift." *Soc Sci & Med* 1991; 32:981–87.

39. Marsh, HW. "Academic Self-Concept: Theory, Measurement, and Research." In Suls, J, editor, *Psychological Perspectives on the Self.* Hillsdale, N.J.: Erlbaum, 1993: 1–26. Marsh, HW, Parker, JW. "Determinants of Student Self-Concept: Is It Better To Be a Relatively Large Fish in a Small Pond Even if You Don't Know How to Swim As Well?" *J Personal Soc Psychol* 1984; 47:213–31.

40. Schwarz, N, Strack, F. "Reports of Subjective Well-Being: Judgmental Processes and Their Methodological Implications." In Kahneman, D, Diener,

E, Schwarz, N, editors, *Well-Being: Foundations of Hedonic Psychology*. New York: Russell-Sage, 1999: 61–84.

41. Strack, F, Schwarz, N, Chassein, B, Kern, D, Wagner, D. "The Salience of Comparison Standards and the Activation of Social Norms: Consequences for Judgments of Happiness and Their Communication." *Brit Journal of Soc Psychol* 1990; 29:303–14.

42. Affleck, G, Tennen, H, Pfeiffer, C, Fifield, J, Rowe, J. "Downward Comparison and Coping with Serious Medical Problems." *Am J Orthopsych* 1987; 57:570–78. Wood, JV, Taylor, SE, Lichtman, RR. "Social Comparison in Adjustment to Breast Cancer." *J Personal Soc Psychol* 1985; 49:1169–83.

43. DeVillis, RF, Holt, K, Renner, BR, Blalock, SJ, Blanchard, LW, Cook, HL, et al. "The Relationship of Social Comparison to Rheumatoid Arthritis Symptoms and Affect." *Basic and Appl Soc Psychol* 1990; 11: 1–18.

44. Strack, F, et al., "The Salience of Comparison Standards."

45. Barsky, AJ. *Worried Sick.*

46. Fitzgerald, FT. "The Tyranny of Health." *New Engl J Med* 1994; 331:196–98.

47. Barsky, AJ. *Worried Sick.*

48. Relman, AS. "The New Medical-Industrial Complex." *New Engl J Med* 1980; 303:963–70.

49. Ibid. Relman, AS. "What Market Values Are Doing to Medicine." *Atlantic Monthly* 1992:99–106. Relman, AS. "The Healthcare Industry: Where Is It Taking Us?" *New Engl J Med* 1991; 325:854–59.

50. Relman, AS. "The New Medical-Industrial Complex."

51. Alper, PA. "Medical Practice in the Competitive Market." *New Engl J Med* 1987; 316:337–39.

52. Gray, "The Selling of Medicine." *Medical Economics* 1986;180.

53. Barsky, AJ. *Worried Sick.*

54. Conrad, P. "Implications of Changing Social Policy for the Medicalization of Deviance." *Contemp Crises* 1980; 4:195–205. Conrad, P. "Medicalization and Social Control." *Ann Rev Sociol* 1992; 18:209–32. Starr, P. *The Social Transformation of American Medicine.* New York: Basic Books, 1982.

55. Oberfield, SE. "Growth Hormone Use in Normal, Short Children—A Plea for Reason." *New Engl J Med* 1999; 340:557–59.

56. Winsten, JA. "Science and the Media: The Boundaries of Truth." *Health Affairs* 1985; 4:5–23.

57. Mann, CC. "Press Coverage: Leaving Out the Big Picture." *Science* 1995; 269:166.

58. Nelkin, D. *Selling Science: How the Press Covers Science and Technology.* New York, NY: WH Freeman Co., 1995. Jauchem, JR. "Epidemiologic Studies of Elec-

tric and Magnetic Fields and Cancer: A Case Study of Distortions by the Media." *J Clin Epidemiol* 1992; 45:1137–42.

59. Relman, AS. "What Market Values Are Doing to Medicine."

60. Christenson, M, Inguanzo, JM. "Smart Consumers Present a Marketing Challenge." *Hospitals* 1989; 63: 42–43.

61. Relman, AS. "The New Medical-Industrial Complex."

62. Grann, D. "Stalking Dr. Steere." *New York Times* 2001 Jun 17:52–57.

63. Treaster, JB. "Rise in Insurance Forces Hospitals to Shutter Wards." *New York Times* 2002 Aug 25:Section 1, Page 1.

Chapter 3

1. Pennebaker, JW. *The Psychology of Physical Symptoms*. New York: Springer-Verlag, 1982.

2. Levine, JD, Gordon, NC, Smith, R, Fields, HL. "Post-Operative Pain: Effect of Extent of Injury and Attention." *Brain Res* 1982; 234:500–04.

Chapter 4

1. Wheeler, EO, Williamson, CR, Cohen, ME. "Heart Scare, Heart Surveys, and Iatrogenic Heart Disease." *JAMA* 1958; 167:1096–102.

2. Thomas, L. *The Lives of a Cell.* New York: Bantam Books, 1975:100.

Chapter 5

1. Pennebaker, JW. *The Psychology of Physical Symptoms.*

2. Beecher, HK. "Relationship of Significance of Wound to Pain Experienced." *JAMA* 1956; 161: 1609–13.

3. Minuchin, S, Rosman, B, Baker, L. *Psychosomatic Families: Anorexia Nervosa in Context.* Cambridge: Harvard University Press, 1978.

Chapter 6

1. Sharpe, M, Hawton, K, Simkin, S, Surawy, C, Hackmann, A, Klimes, I, et al. "Cognitive Behavior Therapy for the Chronic Fatigue Syndrome: A Randomized Clinical Trial." *BMJ* 1996; 312:22–26. Mayou, R, Bass, C, Sharpe, M. *Treatment of Functional Somatic Symptoms.* Oxford: Oxford Univ. Press, 1995.

2. Lucock, MP, Morley, S, White, C, Peake, MD. "Responses of Consecutive Patients to Reassurance After Gastroscopy: Results of a Self-Administered Questionnaire Survey." *Br Med J* 1997; 315:572–75. Channer, KS, James, MA, Papouchado, M, Rees, JR. "Failure of a Negative Exercise Test to Reassure Patients with Chest Pain." *Quart J Med* 1987; 63:315–22.

3.   Myers, MG, Cairns, JA, Singer, J. "The Consent Form as a Possible Cause of Side Effects." *Clin Pharmacol Ther* 1987; 42:250–53.

Chapter 7

1.   Pennebaker, JW. *The Psychology of Physical Symptoms.*

2.   Pennebaker, JW, Beall, SK. "Confronting a Traumatic Event: Toward an Understanding of Inhibition and Disease." *J Abnorm Psychol* 1986; 95:274–81.

3.   Kelley, JE, Lumley, MA, Leisen, JCC. "Health Effects of Emotional Disclosure in Rheumatioid Arthrits Patients." *Health Psychol* 1997; 16:331–40. Smyth, JM, Stone, AA, Hurewitz, A, Kaell, A. "Effects of Writing about Stressful Experiences on Symptom Reduction in Patients with Asthma or Rheumatoid Arthritis: A Randomized Trial." *JAMA* 1999; 281: 1304–09.

4.   Smyth, JM. "Written Emotional Expression Effect Sizes, Outcome Types, and Moderating Variables." *J Consult Clin Psychol* 1998; 66:174–84.

Chapter 8

1.   Vaillant, GE. *Aging Well.* New York: Little, Brown & Company, 2002.

Chapter 9

1. Farshchi, HR, Taylor, MA, and MacDonald, IA. "Regular Meal Frequency Creates More Appropriate Insulin Sensitivity and Lipid Profiles Compared with Irregular Meal Frequency in Healthy Lean Women." *Eur J Clin Nut* 2004; 58:1071–77.

2. Jenkins, DJ, Wolever, TM, Vuksan, V, Brighenti, F, Cunnane, SC, Rao, AV, Jenkins, AL, Buckley, G, Patten, R, Singer, W. "Nibbling Versus Gorging: Metabolic Advantages of Increased Meal Frequency." *New Engl J M* 1991; 321:929–34.

3. Iwao, S, Mori, K, and Sato, Y. "Effects of Meal Frequency on Body Composition During Weight Control in Boxers." *Scan J Med and Science in Sports* 1996; 6:265–72.

4. Data presented by Dr. Mark Pereira of Harvard Medical School at the American Heart Association's 43rd Annual Conference, March 5–8, 2003, Miami.

5. Butrin, R, et al. *Taking a Closer Look at Phytochemicals.* American Institute of Cancer Research, 2003.

6. Stoll, AL, Severus, E, Freeman, MP, Rueter, S, et al. "Omega-3 Fatty Acids in Bipolar Disorder: A Preliminary Double-Blind, Placebo-Controlled Trial." *Arch Gen Psych* 1999; 56:407–12.

7. "AHRQ Evidence Reports Confirm That Fish Oil Helps Fight Heart Disease." Press release, April 22,

2004. Agency for Healthcare Research and Quality, Rockville, MD.

8.   Harvard School of Public Health. "Fats and Cholesterol: Research from the Ongoing Nurses' Health Study at Harvard Medical School." At www.hsph. harvard.edu/nutritionsource/fats.html.

9.   Landers, SJ. "Alphabet Overload." *AMA News* 2004; 47: 25–26.

10. *President's Council on Physical Fitness and Sports Research Digest.* March 2004, Series 5, No. 1.

11. Blair, SN, Kohl, HW, III, Barlow, CE, Paffenbager, RS, Jr, Gibbons, LW, Macera, CA. "Changes in Physical Fitness and All-Cause Mortality: A Prospective Study of Healthy and Unhealthy Men." *JAMA* 1995; 273:1093–98.

12. Fletcher, et al. "Statement on Exercise: Benefits and Recommendations for Physical Activity Programs for All Americans." *Circulation* 1996; 94:857–62.

13. Tran, ZV, Weltman, A. "Differential Effects of Exercise on Serum Lipid and Lipoprotein Levels Seen with Changes in Body Weight: A Meta Analysis." *JAMA* 1985; 254:919–24.

14. Centers for Disease Control. "Strength Training Among Adults aged > 65 Years, United States, 2001." *MMWR Weekly* 2002; 53:25–28.

15. At www.cdc.gov/nccdphp/dnpa/physical/growing_ stronger/why.htm.

16. Ibid.

17. Ibid.

18. *President's Council on Physical Fitness and Sports Research Digest.* June 2000, Series 3, No. 10.

Chapter 10

1. Illich, I. *Medical Nemesis.* New York: Bantam Books, 1976.

2. Ibid.

3. Barsky, AJ. *Worried Sick.*

4. Ibid.

Index ———————————————————